OCTAVIA WILBERFORCE

OCTAVIA WILBERFORCE

THE AUTOBIOGRAPHY OF A PIONEER WOMAN DOCTOR

Edited by Pat Jalland

CASSELL

Cassell Publishers Limited
Artillery House, Artillery Row
London SW1P 1RT

Copyright © Pat Jalland 1989

The original manuscript of 'The Eighth Child' by
Octavia Wilberforce copyright © Mabel Smith and
the Trustees of Backsettown

First published 1989

Distributed in Australia by
Capricorn Link (Australia) Pty Ltd
PO Box 665, Lane Cove, NSW 2066

British Library Cataloguing in Publication Data

Wilberforce, Octavia
Octavia Wilberforce
1. Great Britain. Medicine. Biographies
I. Title II. Jalland, Pat
610'.92'4

ISBN 0-304-32230-X

Typeset in 11/13½ pt Garamond by Input Typesetting
Printed in Great Britain
by Mackays of Chatham

PICTURE ACKNOWLEDGEMENTS

Backsettown Trust; Camera Press;
Dean and Chapter of Westminster;
East Sussex County Library;
Evening Argus, Brighton; Marjorie Baker;
Mary Evans Picture Library; Royal Free Hospital, London;
Sussex Express and County Herald; Wellcome Institute Library, London;
West Sussex Record Office.

CONTENTS

ACKNOWLEDGEMENTS AND NOTE ON EDITORIAL POLICY

I wish to thank Mabel Smith and the Trustees of Backsettown, copyright owners of Octavia Wilberforce's 'The Eighth Child', for their permission to publish this edited version. Mabel Smith's enthusiasm for the project, her encouragement and additional information have been invaluable. She also kindly permitted me to include Octavia's letters to Elizabeth Robins from the Graylingwell Mental Hospital and the Rotunda Hospital, Dublin. Mabel also undertook the search for the photographs used in the book. I am immensely grateful for her friendship and hospitality, and I dedicate this book to her. My thanks are also due to my friend, Dee Cook, and to the helpful librarians at the Fawcett Library for their assistance at the start of this project. Last but not least, I am indebted to Jan Kelly and Genelle Jones for their splendidly efficient work in transferring this manuscript to the word processor.

My chief task as editor was to reduce an unwieldy typescript of 390 pages to half that length. My general policy was to delete long anecdotal passages, lengthy descriptions of holidays and travel, much of the discursive childhood narrative and some material on Elizabeth Robins's later life. Chapters were reduced to twelve, with new titles added; punctuation was corrected and repetition eliminated. Other stylistic details – spelling, hyphenation, numerals, use of capitals, etc. – have been standardised, where appropriate. Two new chapters have been inserted on Octavia's experiences at Graylingwell and Dublin, using her letters to Elizabeth Robins. I decided against inserting three points to indicate omissions, since they would appear so frequently as to interfere with the clarity and flow of the prose. I have endeavoured throughout to remain as faithful as possible to Octavia's original text.

FOR MABEL SMITH

INTRODUCTION
Pat Jalland

Precisely a month before her suicide in 1941, Virginia Woolf asked if she might write a 'portrait' of her friend Octavia Wilberforce. Virginia considered Octavia 'very paintable. That's the sort of woman I most admire – the reticence, the quiet, the power. She's healing the sick by day, and controlling the [wartime] fires by night.' After Virginia's death, Leonard Woolf subsequently encouraged Octavia to write this autobiography. Octavia's four-hundred-page typescript and her letters to Elizabeth Robins came to my attention during a search for the correspondence and diaries of pioneer women doctors. The story of Octavia's life was fascinating in itself, while the material was so clearly also significant for the history of women, the history of feminism and the history of women in medicine.

Leonard Woolf was impressed by 'the fineness and genuineness' of Octavia's character, with its depth and many facets – generous minded but without illusions, complex yet rocklike. He admired Octavia as 'a free soul . . . a remarkable woman . . . her roots were in English history'. Like her friend, Elizabeth Robins, she was a 'through and through individualist; both of them, with great difficulty, with great strength of mind and will, broke away from the fetters of their family and class'.[1] Octavia was a member of the famous Wilberforce family, which revered her great-grandfather, William, emancipator of the slaves, and her grandfather, Samuel, Bishop of Winchester. She struggled for many years to achieve a sense of her own purpose in life. Throughout her childhood and adolescence she was powerfully aware that her birth had been unwelcome to middle-aged parents with seven older children, and she even knew of her mother's attempt to 'get rid of me'. Characteristically, Octavia added, 'but that only gave me my first trial in Persistence.'

Despite the absence of formal education and her parents' lack of interest in her upbringing, Octavia Wilberforce grew up with a surprisingly strong sense of her own identity, even if her role in life was far from clear. She knew from an early stage the qualities she appreciated and the pursuits which were worthwhile. Octavia admired honesty, integrity, humour, zest for life, determination and strength of character – qualities which she herself possessed in good measure. Presentation at Court in 1907 failed to impress her, and she was relieved to return to 'my rose growing, my Sussex friends and my golf'. She was already confident by the age of twenty that her chief aim in life was not to make a 'good' marriage, like her sisters, but 'to mean something in the world'. She had the self-knowledge to reject a highly eligible suitor at the age of twenty-three, despite intense family pressure and the recognition that prospects for upper-class spinsters were poor. She also possessed the strength of mind and will to persevere in medical studies despite constant ridicule and resistance from her family, and despite all academic obstacles.

Octavia's autobiography and correspondence have considerable value for the history of women and of feminism. Her early life story illuminates the limited opportunities and inadequate education of many upper- and upper-middle-class girls right up to 1914. It also illustrates the tough struggle against rigid parental authority necessary for such girls who were sufficiently unusual and independent to prefer a career to a suitable marriage. Octavia's early history underlines the limits to the achievements of 'first wave' feminism; only a supreme effort saved her from becoming a 'hand slave to family life', caring for elderly parents, or allowing them to pressure her into a marriage which repelled her. On several occasions she compared women's struggle for emancipation with the campaign of her great-grandfather, William Wilberforce, to free the slaves; and William's example encouraged her in her own fight for freedom. At moments of personal success she visited Westminster Abbey to tell the good news to William Wilberforce, 'sitting benignly in his chair'.

Octavia Wilberforce's feminism was demonstrated through her life and her work as a doctor. She was sympathetic and supportive towards the activist feminist campaigns of her friends Elizabeth Robins and Lady Rhondda; they in turn appreciated that Octavia was contributing to the progress of women in the medical profession, as well as helping her women patients, and using her own talents in the best way possible. Octavia Wilberforce's feminism was influenced by the ideas of Elizabeth Robins, especially in the early years. Both friends believed that women needed identities and destinies of their own, instead of existing primarily in relationship to men. But they must first win economic independence to allow emotional and intellectual freedom. Octavia's medical career enhanced her practical understanding of the restrictions on women's lives, and inspired illuminating comments on both the problems and their possible causes. For example, her work at Graylingwell Mental Hospital led her to analyse the dangers of emotional and financial dependence. She was concerned to discover that such a large proportion of female mental patients were former servants, governesses and housewives: 'Were slaves ever mad? What about its being mentally unhealthy to be the underdog?' Octavia thought that research into such causes of female madness would illuminate the more general problems of the female condition.[2]

Octavia's autobiography sheds new light on the feminist campaign and its leaders during the two years immediately following the concession of the vote to women over thirty in 1918. Through Elizabeth Robins, Octavia became friendly with Lady Rhondda, who launched an influential feminist periodical called *Time and Tide* in 1920, 'to enable women's voices to be heard in the political forum' now they had gained the vote and to remedy some of the deficiencies in women's political education.[3] Octavia was busily preparing for uncongenial Surgery examinations at the time, but she saw a good deal of Lady Rhondda, particularly because Elizabeth Robins was on the original board of women directors of *Time and Tide*. Lady Rhondda 'was full of ideas about the position and potential power of women in the world', which she expounded to Octavia during lengthy discussions.

During Octavia's difficult struggle to become a doctor, she frequently found peace to study and recover at Backsettown, Elizabeth Robins's beautiful fifteenth-century farmhouse in Sussex. This subsequently gave her the idea to use Backsettown as a convalescent home to provide a 'rest pause' for overworked professional women and mothers with heavy domestic responsibilities. The aim was to restore normal vigour to over-fatigued women through rest in congenial surroundings, a good vitamin-enriched diet, and ultra-violet radiation when necessary.[4] The project began in 1927, aided by Octavia's efforts to produce clean milk from her own tuberculin-tested herd of Jersey cows. Despite continuing financial problems the number of patients increased after the war, and after her retirement, until her death in 1963, Octavia devoted all her time to the women convalescents and to farming at Backsettown.

Octavia Wilberforce's autobiography and correspondence are also important for the history of women in medicine. Octavia was one of the second generation of pioneer women doctors, but was old enough to encounter many of the same difficulties as the first generation. Her memoir and correspondence provide a rich source for the experience of women in medicine, a field where good primary sources, such as correspondence and diaries, are rare.

The story of the leading pioneers of the first generation of women doctors is well known, but a brief summary will serve to place Octavia's experience in context. Elizabeth Blackwell was the first woman to have her name entered on the medical register in 1859, but only after an American training. The second pioneer, Elizabeth Garrett, succeeded in passing the examination of the London Society of Apothecaries in 1865, before the Society changed its constitution to exclude female candidates from their examination. The important campaign for women in medicine began when Sophia Jex-Blake and several sister students survived four gruelling years of medical study at Edinburgh University only to be told in 1873 that, as women, they could not be examined for their degrees. The bold response of Sophia Jex-Blake was to establish the London School of Medicine for Women, which opened in Brunswick Square with fourteen students in 1874. After two years of intensive campaigning, Parliament passed a law permitting all medical bodies to admit women to their examinations. The London School of Medicine for Women was formally placed on the list of registered medical schools, and agreement was reached with the Royal Free Hospital in 1877 for the women students to obtain clinical training there. Student numbers increased from about sixty in 1883 to more than three hundred in 1902, when Elizabeth Garrett Anderson resigned as Dean.

Despite the achievements of the first generation of pioneers, the campaign for the general acceptance of women doctors in England was still being fought at the outbreak of the First World War. It was not until the war that the numbers of women applying to study medicine increased to any extent, while medical education continued to be rigidly segregated according to gender. When Octavia Wilberforce first approached the London School of Medicine for Women in 1913 for information, she learned that there were nine hundred qualified women as against thirty thousand men. Most of these female doctors were obliged to work abroad, especially in India, where high-caste Indian women were not allowed to consult male doctors. Trained women who remained in Britain were engaged chiefly in public work because so much prejudice still existed against women in private practice, especially in small country towns.

Octavia Wilberforce encountered the same arguments against medical women which assailed the first generation of pioneers. Her family argued vehemently that medicine was 'unsexing' for women, that they lacked the physical stamina for it, and would starve after the training, since it was impossible for them to make a living. Octavia was told that she would waste the best years of her youth on the training, she would lose all her friends and would wreck her chance of becoming a good wife and mother. She was sternly informed that she would do more good by marrying for money or staying at home to look after her parents. Her father's opposition was so extreme as to 'disclaim any further interest' in Octavia as a daughter, to refuse to pay the £1000 needed for seven years' medical training and living expenses, and to cut her out of his will. She was entirely dependent on the financial support of friends like Elizabeth Robins and Sydney Buxton for her fees and frugal accommodation, living in London for seven years on £100 a year. Whenever she visited her family in Sussex she was subjected to 'every kind of abuse', and the 'anti-doctoring, anti-women' stream of harassment continued until she qualified.

Octavia Wilberforce suffered from her class as well as her gender in her struggle to become a doctor. As Leonard Woolf noted: 'In those days in Sussex, country house young ladies did not become doctors; they married and bred more young ladies.'[5] Octavia's upbringing as a young lady was more deficient than most, due to parental neglect; she received only one year of formal schooling, apart from sporadic instruction in History, Literature and Music from occasional tutors. The minimum entrance requirement for medical school was the London matriculation examination in five subjects at the same sitting, including Latin and Mathematics, of which she was almost totally ignorant. Despite immense effort and special coaching, she struggled against seven failures in matriculation from 1911 to 1915, when she finally passed the Cambridge Senior Higher Local examination instead, as it was 'more coachable'. Her mind was untrained when she embarked on her studies in 1911 at the age of twenty-three, and she suffered accordingly. Octavia later attributed the happiness of her life to the persistence and discipline required to overcome these obstacles of lack of money and formal education. She acquired a sense of proportion and zest for life: 'one has been conditioned to plumb the depths and afterwards how greatly has one learned to appreciate the heights.'[6]

Octavia's account of her prolonged medical training at the London School of Medicine for Women from 1913 to 1920 is illuminating both for her own tough struggle and for the advances made by medical women during the war. Wartime conditions helped to break down the barriers separating male and female students and to reduce male medical prejudice against women doctors and students. Octavia contributed to this advance. She was determined to prove that women could work on equal terms with male doctors, 'to help consolidate women's position in medicine', and prove women just as capable as the men students. Octavia did her clinical training in 1917–18 at St Mary's Hospital, Paddington, which only accepted a few women students 'as an experiment' because potential male students were away fighting in the war. 'It mattered enormously that the women allowed to invade such a male-bound, prejudiced hospital' should make a good impression. She was 'blissfully happy' as clinical clerk to Dr Wilfred Harris, who considered her a good diagnostician. Octavia spent two years on the wards at St Mary's Hospital from 1918 to 1920, when returned soldiers had to become accustomed to women as colleagues and students.

Octavia's first paid job after she qualified was that of House Physician to Dr Harris at St Mary's, followed by Assistant Medical Officer at Paddington Infirmary. She longed to become a consultant in London, but this was too risky and expensive: 'My determination was to be self-supporting and I was more than anxious to convince my family of my success.' So Octavia chose the alternative of putting up a brass plate in Brighton, which was also a risky enterprise for a woman, though less so than consultancy. At the age of thirty-four she bought a house in Brighton with loans from women friends and worked hard to establish her practice. In time she was also appointed a full Physician at the New Sussex Hospital, staffed only by women for the treatment of female patients. Octavia shared the view of its founder, Louisa Martindale, that there was an urgent need for women to be treated by members of their own sex.[7] Octavia found medical practice 'a life of great rewards . . . a life which gives an independence of spirit which can rarely be achieved in family and personal relationships'.

The two chapters on 'Midwifery in Dublin, 1918' and 'A Mental Hospital in 1920' provide fascinating insights into midwifery and mental health immediately after the First World War. Both experiences are revealed through Octavia's daily letters to Elizabeth Robins, which give a detailed, vivid account of aspects of hospital life and medical work of interest to her non-medical friend. In 1918 Octavia Wilberforce did four weeks' practical midwifery training at the Rotunda Hospital in Dublin, considered the best in the world at the time. Octavia's account is particularly interesting because it describes midwifery in the Dublin slums in the period immediately prior to the more general hospitalisation of childbirth. She agreed with the Dublin doctors that the risk of sepsis was too great in poor, over-crowded homes, but it was not easy to persuade women to go to hospital. At first Octavia considered midwifery 'horrid, filthy and messy', but quickly found it a gratifying branch of medicine, with 'such quick results for your trouble'. Her detailed descriptions of individual cases provide valuable insights into practical midwifery in Dublin two decades before the general use of antibiotics.

Octavia was also a keen observer of the relationships between the different hierarchical levels of medical staff, especially where the issue of gender was involved. She was critical of another student named Bellows who drew attention to her sex by flirting with senior male medical staff. Even worse, Bellows concluded an argument with a male doctor over a tragic case involving a baby's death at birth: 'I wish you men could have babies for a year or two.' Octavia was furious: 'If you go in for Medicine you've simply got to forget the differences in sex, else you'll make the whole work impossible. I can't tell you how damaging to women's doing Medicine is a remark as personal as that.' By contrast, Octavia wanted male doctors and surgeons to forget they were working with a woman, particularly the older and more distrustful males: 'We've got to consolidate our position as *medical* colleagues, and not go sliding back into "girls" and personalities.'

This volume is also important for its unusual perspective on the life of Elizabeth Robins, and for its insights into the nature of female friendships. Elizabeth Robins entered Octavia Wilberforce's life in 1909, and while her later years are described in the autobiography, her more famous earlier career requires some introduction here. Dale Spender has recently described Elizabeth Robins as 'an exciting and currently relevant personality.

. . . She was such a superb writer, and her politics invite such enthusiastic response today.'⁸ Elizabeth Robins was an American, born into a wealthy gentry family in Kentucky in 1862. Leonard Woolf recalled her:

> . . . a small, beautiful, mercurial woman, she had, in a very high degree, that inexplicable and indefinable quality, personal charm. She was as quick and elusive as quicksilver and at the same time amazingly tenacious. Most people fell in love with her, or at least were charmed and dominated by her. She was a famous actress and a brilliant writer.⁹

Elizabeth shocked her family at the age of sixteen by declaring that she intended to become an actress, and she joined the Boston Museum Stock Company despite her father's disapproval. She played 380 parts with them in 1883–4, and later toured America with Edwin Booth's troupe. Early in her American acting career, she was induced to marry an American actor, George Parks, because he otherwise threatened suicide. This ill-fated match taught her extreme caution in subsequent relationships, especially since he drowned himself a few years later in the Charles River, dressed in a medieval suit of armour.

When she went to England in 1888, initially en route to a Norwegian holiday, she met Oscar Wilde, who introduced her to the English theatre world and encouraged her to try her fortunes on the London stage. West End theatres were largely controlled by male actor-managers who chose plays to display their own talents, so that Elizabeth found her roles unchallenging and melodramatic. In 1891 another disenchanted actress, Marion Lea, suggested that they should produce and co-star in the controversial Ibsen drama, *Hedda Gabler*. This ambitious and courageous enterprise involved finding funds, gaining production rights and persuading audiences to attend in the face of powerful opposition. *Hedda Gabler* had an unprecedented seven-week run for an 'experimental', scandalous play and Elizabeth won great acclaim for her superb performance as Hedda. In the 1890s Ibsen was the spearhead of the campaign against traditional drama and Elizabeth Robins played a vital role in the Ibsen movement. She boldly continued to produce the plays of Ibsen alone after her partner's marriage, establishing herself as a talented actress-manageress, producing and performing in her own independent productions. She introduced five Ibsen dramas to sceptical English audiences and helped to translate them as soon as they appeared. Her financial position was always precarious because her experimental theatre brought in little money and other directors were reluctant to cast her in more popular conventional roles. [10]

As a beautiful, single actress, Elizabeth Robins encountered some difficulties in maintaining relationships with male colleagues on a purely business basis. After her success as Hedda Gabler in 1891 she was pursued by several suitors, but the most persistent of these was William Heinemann, the Ibsen publisher. After a year of rejecting his insistent marriage proposals, she finally aimed a pistol at him to discourage further pursuit. This melodramatic tactic was less effective in discouraging the unwanted amorous attentions of George Bernard Shaw. When Shaw finally accepted her puritanical message, he cast more amenable actresses in his plays. [11] Elizabeth Robins was more ambivalent about her relationships with William Archer and Henry James because she found them more sympathetic, and therefore they posed a greater threat to her independence. The theatre critic and Ibsen translator, William Archer, was a friend and ally of Elizabeth's, but she fought to check her feelings for him:

> Even W.A. my strongest anchor to good, good cheer and wholesome activity is coming to demand too much of me of time and regard. It would not be hard for me to love this man not wisely but too well and I must guard my poor life against a curse like that. For soon after I had acknowledged him the one being in the world for me he would possess the supremest power to pain me, and unconsciously and inevitably he would use his power. Not that he would *wish* to . . . but he would be as helpless as I. [12]

Elizabeth Robins and Henry James became close friends after

she played the heroine in his play, *The American*, in 1891. She called their relationship a 'participation' in theatre and friendship, and she may have been in love with James.[13]

Her career as an actress and producer came abruptly to a close in 1898 when she courageously departed for the Klondyke during the gold rush. She left London at the height of her personal fame on the London stage, in search of her beloved younger brother, whose fate concerned her after a prolonged silence. Most friends thought her misguided to go to the Klondyke to look for Raymond, but W.T. Stead advanced the funds for the expedition. After many trials and tribulations she found her brother ill and nursed him back to health, but she was struck with typhoid in Alaska, leaving her an invalid for some years afterwards.

Elizabeth Robins later told Dame Sybil Thorndike that she left the stage while still in her prime because she found little in the theatre world that was satisfying as an entire way of life.[14] She may also have been influenced by the lack of financial stability in her theatre career, given her concern about women's need for economic independence. In any case, she had already turned to her second career as a writer during the 1890s, producing three novels under the pen name of C.E. Raimond. Her first novel, *George Mandeville's Husband*, was acclaimed by the critics in 1894 as showing great promise. The authorship of her first three novels was the subject of considerable speculation, but they were accepted as the work of a man. Her identity was exposed by accident in 1898 after she published *The Open Question*, which attracted considerable attention and placed her novels 'high in the ranks of contemporary fiction'. Her next book, *The Magnetic North*, which appeared in 1903, told the story of her adventures in the Klondyke and 'remains probably her finest literary work'.[15]

Elizabeth Robins was a committed feminist from her early years in the theatre. She became a member of the militant suffrage campaign, the Women's Social and Political Union, during the decade before the First World War. Her 1907 play, *Votes for Women*, provided valuable propaganda and a slogan for the cause, while her 1913 book, *Where Are You Going To?*, condemned the white slave traffic. Of her many subsequent books, *Ancilla's Share* in 1924 provided the most complete analysis of her feminist views, reinforced by her articles in *Time and Tide*. She believed that many means were necessary to secure women's emancipation, and that the campaign for women's rights must not end just because the female vote was won. She attacked male power and the subordination of women, appealing particularly for women's economic independence, which was the vital prerequisite for all other forms of freedom.[16]

It is easy to understand why the young Octavia Wilberforce found Elizabeth Robins so fascinating. The relationship with the American actress and writer was the most important in Octavia's life, lasting from 1909 until Elizabeth Robins's death in 1952. They met when Octavia was twenty-one and Elizabeth forty-seven: 'It was a turning point in my life . . . hero worship at first sight.' This new friendship transformed and greatly influenced Octavia's life. Elizabeth Robins challenged Octavia to seek the education she never had, and subsequently encouraged her to become a doctor, despite intense family opposition. Octavia wrote to Elizabeth Robins in 1911: 'You made me think that I was an individual . . . You are the one being whom I have come to care for with all the concentrated, bottled up affection of twenty-three years.' Five years later, Octavia asked her friend if she might regard her 'as my adopted mother', though by 1918 Octavia considered herself 'more than a daughter'. Their relationship altered after Octavia qualified in 1920: 'Her association with me over those long struggling years was essentially a maternal one – protective, far-seeing, ambitious for my success.' After qualification the focus shifted and Octavia's devotion to Elizabeth Robins became more adult and equal. When Octavia started her practice in Brighton in 1923 Elizabeth Robins continued to write novels from her London base, joining Octavia in Brighton for weekends, holidays and, as her health declined, increasingly also for nursing. Octavia believed that married women with many family ties and responsibilities could not easily become first-class doctors, whereas her own concentration on medicine was essentially strengthened by her love for Elizabeth Robins.

Recent research into the nature of female friendships in the nineteenth century helps to explain the relationship between the two women. Carroll Smith-Rosenberg has argued that the Victorian domestic ideology which confined middle- and upper-class women to the domestic sphere led to the emotional segregation of women and men, and generated a sense of intimacy and sisterhood among women. Women friends chiefly provided comfort and companionship through adolescence, courtship and marriage, as well as through pregnancies, sickness, spinsterhood and death. Relationships between women in the nineteenth century were complex and diverse, traversing a wide range of feelings and behaviour, from the long-lived and platonic dedication of sisters and beloved friends, to the romantic enthusiasms of adolescents, and the more passionate love of some mature women. Nineteenth-century women's friendships were characterised by 'closeness, freedom of emotional expression, and uninhibited physical contact', while the taboos were placed rather on premarital heterosexual relationships. Female friendships were socially acceptable until twentieth-century sexologists created a dichotomy between relationships categorised as either normal or deviant, and developed new cultural taboos to facilitate the process.[17]

The 'female world of love and ritual' evidently declined in the early twentieth century, though it seems likely that it survived among that minority of independent women who deliberately chose not to marry. As an American feminist, Dr Clelia Mosher, wrote in her journal in 1919:

There is a kind of Friendship which may exist among women where their individual interests are so merged, that each has for the other the same vital interest in the other's success as the mother has in her daughter's affairs. . . . It has all the wonderful community interest one finds in ideal marriage and only differs in the absence of the physical relationship. It is emotionally satisfying.

But she concluded: 'One seldom sees it', for it is 'only possible to a very high type of woman, spiritually and intellectually.'[18] It may have been rare by 1919, but it certainly existed between Elizabeth Robins and Octavia Wilberforce, in precisely that sense defined by Clelia Mosher. In later life Octavia confided in Mabel Smith that 'a lasting and deeply-loving relationship was entirely possible without sex', and that she knew of two such friendships.[19]

Elizabeth Robins was essentially a woman of the nineteenth century, who deeply appreciated the values of close female friendships, especially that she formed from the 1890s with Florence Bell, wife of Sir Hugh Bell, a wealthy ironmaster. By contrast, experience had taught her that male friendships, particularly if they led to marriage or had the potential to do so, would 'possess the supremest power to pain me'. Therefore she took care not to allow her affection for William Archer to tempt her into a second marriage, which might stifle her brilliant creativity and threaten her personal autonomy. So Elizabeth Robins maintained her independence, while her devoted friendship with Lady Bell continued until the latter's death in 1930, reinforced by regular correspondence and several lengthy visits each year to the Bells' Yorkshire home. Elizabeth Robins celebrated victory in November 1918 with a brief note to Florence Bell: 'My dearest: I've felt ever since the peace signals sounded that I wanted to make *my* sign to the particular one of the nation who has meant most to me all these years. Beloved, I embrace you.'[20] Elizabeth Robins and Octavia corresponded in similar style, particularly after their friendship attained a more equal basis in 1920. Their affectionate terms of endearment are alien to most later twentieth-century readers, and care is needed in interpretation.[21]

Octavia Wilberforce was twenty-one when she met the famous actress in 1909. Her home life had been particularly sheltered, with little parental affection or interest, no siblings close to her own age to play with and no formal schooling to encourage friendships. Octavia made two good friends among girls in neighbouring families, but she had experienced no romantic attachments by the age of twenty-one. Several references in her autobiography suggest that Octavia Wilberforce was reserved and physically undemonstrative. Two episodes described in detail in the memoir are particularly revealing about her attitudes towards male and female relationships, marriage and homosexuality. First, in 1911 a personal crisis was caused by an unwelcome marriage proposal from Charles Buxton, son of Sydney Buxton, a Liberal Cabinet Minister. Octavia's family pressured her to accept this eligible suitor, fearing that 'female friendships' would discourage her from making a good marriage. When she rejected Charlie Buxton's proposal, Octavia was repelled by the physical prospect of marriage:

> I suddenly felt so revolted at what it all meant from *my* point of view. I was so staggered at the horror of such thoughts that to prevent the sleeve of his coat touching mine I walked in the ditch. If I have ever grown up it was at that moment.

She felt reduced 'to the same level as an animal' by his 'craving for possession'. The episode convinced her she was not 'cut out' for marriage – 'the very thought of it makes me shudder'. She would rather be a golf professional or a 'sweaty cook' than a kept wife. This crisis illustrates Octavia's innocence, immaturity and inexperience at the age of twenty-three. It also shows how powerful her revulsion was at the 'physical prospect' of marriage, which evidently overwhelmed her by its horror. She was repelled at the prospect of being possessed and therefore dependent.

The second significant episode took place five years later. Octavia was then living in a London hostel with 'women of different ages in many different walks of life', none of whom were likely to interfere with her liberty – preferring this to a 'wholly student atmosphere'. She was intensely resentful and disturbed by the homosexual harassment of a fellow student, though she did not recognise its nature at the time. Octavia was twenty-eight 'but of homosexuality I knew nothing'. She became terrified of the girl's 'obsession', which she considered 'ugly, alarming and unhinged'. 'The guarded explanations of what I had taken to be mental derangement came as a considerable shock to my innocence.' Octavia then became aware of the dichotomy between normal and deviant behaviour. She recognised that many girls had firm friendships which were both 'normal and healthy', like her own with Phyllis and Joan. Possibly for the first time she wondered about the precise category of her friendship with Elizabeth Robins, because during this same period she asked if she might look upon her as an adopted mother. By 1920 Octavia no longer worried about it, as she gained in confidence and experience, and absorbed Elizabeth Robins's more flexible Victorian attitudes towards female friendships.

Finally, Octavia's autobiography is valuable for the new light it sheds on Virginia Woolf's tragic last year. In May 1940 Virginia Woolf completed her biography of Roger Fry; as so often happened, the stimulation of writing a book was followed by serious depression. Octavia Wilberforce became friendly with the Woolfs in 1940, initially because she sent them regular contributions of Jersey milk and cream from her herd. Octavia enjoyed the intellectual stimulation of her visits to Virginia and admired that 'heavenly agility of mind'; Virginia, in turn, respected in Octavia 'the reticence, the quiet, the power' and envied her practical, worthwhile profession and her touch with reality. Virginia decided to write a 'living portrait' of Octavia, and their discussions on this project were mutually revealing. Virginia confided her fear that she had lost the art of writing, and her terror that the Second World War would stimulate another bout of madness, just as the First had done. She confessed that she was 'feeling desperate – depressed to the lowest depths', and felt particularly useless in wartime. She talked a good deal about her earlier years, and the burden of her father's excessive 'emotional claims' after her mother's death: 'that, I think, has accounted for many of the wrong things in my life.' Octavia concluded that she was desperate, scared, and 'haunted by her father'.

The day before Virginia's suicide in 1941 she agreed to Leonard's desperate appeal that she should seek Octavia's professional help; after a physical examination the two women discussed Virginia's fears at length, especially her anxiety that the past would recur. Next day, Leonard's news of Virginia's suicide shocked and saddened Octavia, who deeply regretted her inability to avert the tragedy. Octavia and Leonard consoled each other by a lengthy discussion of Virginia's life, her brilliant mind and her terrible mental affliction. Octavia concluded that it was impossible to maintain Virginia's sanity while war continued: 'without war I'm sure I could have helped and completely saved her.' The short friendship between the two women ended tragically and only a few lines survive of Virginia's 'living portrait' of Octavia. However, Octavia consoled herself with the knowledge that her visits helped Virginia to keep 'the Beast at bay' and brought a measure of tranquillity to a deeply troubled mind. Those visits also encouraged Octavia to feel that the story of her own life might be of interest and value to others. In a sense this book begins with Virginia Woolf's death, and is in part a tribute to Virginia's belief in the power of words to illuminate our lives.

NOTES

Quotations without a reference are taken from the main text.

[1] Leonard Woolf, 'Octavia Wilberforce', in *Backsettown, Elizabeth Robins and Octavia Wilberforce*, published for private circulation, 1952, pp. 29–31.

[2] For contemporary research see e.g. Elaine Showalter, *The Female Malady: Women, Madness and English Culture, 1830–1980*, Virago, 1987; Jill Julius Matthews, *Good and Mad Women*, Allen and Unwin, 1984.

[3] See Dale Spender, *Time and Tide Wait for No Man*, Pandora Press, 1984, esp. pp. 4–6.

[4] *Backsettown, Elizabeth Robins and Octavia Wilberforce*, pp. 9–20.

[5] L. Woolf, 'Octavia Wilberforce', p. 30.

[6] Typescripts of Octavia Wilberforce's speeches on 'The Birth of the National Health Service' and 'How to Prepare for Retirement', deposited in the Fawcett Library, London.

[7] Octavia Wilberforce, 'Notes of a talk given under the auspices of the British Council to a group of foreign professional women visiting this country', 1949, Fawcett Library.

[8] Dale Spender, *Time and Tide*, p. 46.

[9] L. Woolf, 'Octavia Wilberforce,' p. 29.

[10] Gay Gibson Cima, 'Elizabeth Robins: the Genesis of an Independent Manageress', *Theatre Survey, XXI*, no. 2 (November, 1980), pp. 145–163. The brief section on Robins's theatre career is based on this useful article. See also Robins, *Both Sides of the Curtain*, 1940.

[11] Cima, 'Elizabeth Robins', pp. 154–8. See also Robins, *Theatre and Friendship: Letters of Henry James*, 1932.

[12] Quoted in Cima, 'Elizabeth Robins', p. 163 (from diary entry, 5 November 1891, Fales Library, New York University).

[13] Edwin Clark, 'Henry James and the Actress', *The Pacific Spectator*, III, no. 1, winter 1949, pp. 86, 91.

[14] Dame Sybil Thorndike, 'Elizabeth Robins as I Knew Her', BBC talk, 6 July 1952, in *Backsettown, Elizabeth Robins and Octavia Wilferforce*, pp. 21–7.

[15] 'Elizabeth Robins', *The Times* obituary, 9 May 1952.

[16] See the excellent commentary on Elizabeth Robins's feminist ideas in Spender, *Time and Tide*, pp. 46–51.

[17] Carroll Smith-Rosenberg, 'The Female World of Love and Ritual: Relations between Women in Nineteenth-Century America', in *Disorderly Conduct. Visions of Gender in Victorian America*, Oxford, 1985, pp. 53–76. See also Sheila Jeffreys, *The Spinster and Her Enemies. Feminism and Sexuality 1880–1930*, London, 1985, esp. pp. 102–7.

[18] Quoted by Carl Degler, *At Odds. Women and the Family in America from the Revolution to the Present*, Oxford, 1980, pp. 149–50.

[19] I am indebted to Mabel Smith for this remark, which she still remembers vividly. The two instances mentioned may have been Elizabeth Robins's friendships with Octavia and with Florence Bell.

[20] Included by Octavia Wilberforce in her typescript of 'The Eighth Child'.

[21] Many years later, when Octavia gave Mabel Smith the Graylingwell letters, she insisted the handwritten originals be destroyed after Mabel had typed copies omitting the affectionate endearments. Octavia hated the thought that readers might misinterpret the terms used. These have largely been retained here in the text of the Dublin letters to illustrate the depth of their friendship in its appropriate context.

OCTAVIA WILBERFORCE

I

A HAPHAZARD
UPBRINGING
The Eighth Child
1888–1909

I was born at Lavington [in Sussex] on 8 January 1888. My father, Reginald Garton Wilberforce, was fifty and my mother forty years old when I was born. My father was the second surviving son of Samuel Wilberforce, Bishop of Oxford and later Winchester, and grandson of William Wilberforce.

My father's varied career [began] as an ensign in the 52nd Light Infantry, where he behaved with great gallantry at the siege of Delhi and was third to enter the city. He [then] returned to England, sold his commission and became a clerk in the House of Commons. But the dull routine of the work did not suit him and his father firmly sent him tea planting to make a fortune in India. In 1866 he returned home to find a wife and take her back to India. In 1867 he married my mother, Annie Maria, third daughter of the Honourable Richard Denman. Instead of returning to India he practised at the Parliamentary Bar while my mother was keeping house for my grandfather, the Bishop. Perhaps my mother's happiest period was when she acted as hostess to her beloved father-in-law at Winchester House. It was, I think, the greatest tragedy of her life when he died in 1873. After his death, while bearing five more children, she devoted herself to dealing with his letters and was, I always felt, the final arbiter in the production of the last two volumes of Bishop Samuel Wilberforce's *Life*.

When the Bishop died in 1873 my parents went to live at Lavington [in Sussex, a large, square Georgian dwelling]. After standing unsuccessfully for Parliament my father took up

I

farming in the disastrous agricultural depression of 1879. My mother meanwhile had begun her family with four sons to be followed by four daughters, I being the eighth child. Two of my brothers took holy orders, one became a barrister and the youngest entered the Indian Civil Service and became Judge of the High Court at Lahore.

My mother had an anxious difficult life with four sons to educate, four daughters to bring up and a husband occupied with the management of the estate, and his duties as a magistrate and member of the County Council. Lavington was a big house to run and as it was five miles from the nearest town, Petworth, servants were hard to find for there were no buses at that time. There was little money coming in from the farms so that Beechwood, the smaller dower house near by, had to be let as added source of income.

A series of tenants came to Beechwood and there were constant family conferences [between] my brother John and my mother over the financial situation when they counselled my father as to what he should do. He was never successful with money and was most happy when shooting, golfing, sitting on the Bench, playing any card game or billiards. I never remember seeing him read anything except newspapers, light novels and the lessons in church on Sunday.

The family consisted of four boys, then three girls, then a gap of seven years and I was found to be on the way. It was most inconvenient. Who wants to reopen a nursery after all those years, and the nurse gone? So my mother 'took steps'. Lavington, nestling under the South Downs, was flanked on the south side by the beech-laden, heavily wooded shoulders of the Downs. A slippery chalk track led to the top of the hill [and after reaching the top it was a walk of over four miles to Charlton Forest]. It was a long walk from Lavington for my mother and she decided to take it in the hope that the effort would bring on a miscarriage and so get rid of me. But that only gave me my first trial in Persistence and her walk had no ill results.

There was twenty years between me and my eldest brother. I might have been treated almost as an only child and greatly spoilt, but instead I was allowed to run wild and, with an insatiably enquiring mind, spent an extremely happy childhood.

At an early age Little Ou, my sister, began to try to teach me to read and write. Writing was a huge labour but so long as I was not sat down to it for too long I did not resent the effort. Learning to read was a different matter. I had cunningly realised that as soon as I could read I should be pushed on to other more time-consuming lessons and I meant to stay in control of my own actions for as long as possible. So I pretended to understand much less than I did and with a mind ranging over far more exciting matters, would slowly pick out C A T cat, R A T rat. Then there came a day when Mr Legge, an established family friend, who talked to me as if I were a grown-up when he took me for walks, suggested how nice and independent it would make me when I could read for myself the Blue Fairy Book – or even the Red. And he bought me a copy and read me a story. I loved it!

It was carelessly stupid of me to be caught one day, deep in a book I was reading by myself. 'Good gracious, do you know that child *can* read?' it was reported. I was furious that my secret had been discovered till I realised I was an object of surprised admiration, and when Mr Legge shortly after arrived on his next visit he was delighted by the news. I really had deserved the box of chocolates he always used to bring me as a present. And next time there was the Green Fairy Book as well for me to devour.

One of my four grown-up brothers tried to teach me sums, but I got no grasp of the subject. My brothers teased me mercilessly and enraged I would fly, either to Mrs Rodgers in the kitchen or to Mr Jones, the coachman, in the stables. These were my stalwart allies and could be relied on for understanding, comfort and support. Mrs Rodgers, deft and efficient, also managed both the bread-making and the dairy. The kitchen, larder, scullery and other offices were in the basement. I loved to watch the way Mrs Rodgers handled things. All children are inquisitive but owing to my mind not being clogged with irrelevant educational facts I could cultivate my powers of observation. Occasionally, if Mrs Rodgers was in a good temper, she would let me try to prepare things myself. She often had words with the other servants, especially the footman, when she was blamed for a dish not being sufficiently hot when it arrived on the table. I never remember Mrs Rodgers being angry with me. What Mr Jones or Mrs Rodgers said I accepted as law, whereas orders from other people were a challenge to be evaded if possible.

The question of my lessons began to loom uncomfortably large. I was not to be allowed so much freedom. A fine of 6d was to be imposed whenever I was found in the kitchen (money was tight and my income was an occasional tip and 6d a week).

'Hush! You run into the larder behind the big flour bin, quick!' whispered Mrs Rodgers and she made a great clatter with the poker in the big fire as one of my sisters came into the kitchen.

'Is Miss Tate down here Mrs Rodgers? She's late for her lessons.' ('Tate' was an abbreviation for Octavia.) Mrs Rodgers, with a raised voice and obviously 'put about', shooed out the intruder.

I was encouraged by [my sister] Susan to learn poetry and allowed to make up my own choice of poems either out of the Golden Treasury or from Shakespeare. I learned 'To be or not to be' and went on to 'The quality of mercy', which much appealed to my nature-loving mind. 'Droppeth as the gentle dew from Heaven' seemed to me finely descriptive! But perhaps my highlight was 'Angels and Ministers of grace defend us' – because I had a profound belief in the Devil and Hell.

To my young ears [my mother played the piano] wonderfully. She also composed an oratorio, the *Saga of King Olaf*, as well as songs. But her playing of Chopin waltzes was what entranced me most and I would sit on a small chair listening till I could bear it no longer and felt I must get up and dance about to the compelling rhythm. I seldom had this treat but the music always haunted me and I'd steal off afterwards to some silent place in the garden and mentally listen all over again to as much as I could remember, by heart.

I was determined to play something and the piano was not encouraged. I had a good ear and one day Mr Whitehead, organist of Chichester Cathedral, who came over to help my mother with the orchestration of *King Olaf*, suggested that I might try the violin. I loved the idea, a violin was procured, and I went into Chichester for lessons from him. I felt proudly independent and I was to lunch at the Palace with Uncle Ernest who was then Bishop of Chichester. Mr Whitehead soon realised that I never practised and threatened to give me up as a waste of his time. He was absolutely right. I would be left in a room where my scratchings could not be heard and having tuned the instrument and found I could not at once reproduce any recognisable tune, I became quickly discouraged. I immersed myself in a Dumas or a Walter Scott novel till the allotted time was nearly at an end, when I would be found dutifully practising by the unsuspecting person who came to fetch me for lunch. My music lessons and my enjoyable visits to Chichester soon ceased, and as I supposed they thought I had to be taught something else, I bicycled the five miles into Petworth twice weekly for French lessons.

Other lessons included learning to ride on Patience, the twenty-eight-year-old pony, who had taught all my brothers and sisters. Mr Jones [the coachman] superintended. He taught me to groom, saddle her and bed her down. Mr Jones had strong views about behaviour and one day up on the Downs when Patience had thrown me and galloped home alone rejoicing, I was greatly put about. It was a hot summer's day and my short legs had to bring me down a long way. When safely back I stole into the coach house and unhitched a carriage whip. Patience was contentedly munching hay when I entered the stable. I was just about to give her what I considered a well-deserved thrashing when Mr Jones suddenly appeared. He snatched the whip from my hand and gave me such a talking to that I felt utterly ashamed – 'trying to take advantage of an old friend, and it was your own fault for falling off anyhow,' he said. I owe a lot to Mr Jones.

Mr Legge was a bachelor whom my father had met at the *Cocoa Tree* in London which, I gathered, was a club where men gambled. He had been in a solicitor's office and became a kind of agent to the Lavington estate, which meant he visited us fairly often and always at holiday times. I looked forward to these visits enormously when I was allowed more in the front of the house. I was greatly attached to him and he was certainly very kind to me. He introduced me to Dumas and gave me *Monte Cristo* and *The Three Musketeers*. He was a constant writer in the *Pall Mall Gazette* and the *Illustrated London News*, and he regaled my mother, to whom he was devoted, with all the latest London literary gossip. He was an Egyptologist and went out to Egypt with other archaeologists to dig up mummies and his talk was most exciting for my young ears. He must have been a source of great diversion and interest to my mother; he used to bring her the latest French novels, and encouraged her musical composition. He also helped her with the sorting out of the Wilberforce letters and her publication of the *Private Papers of William Wilberforce*.

[In the 1890s] my father had been induced to invest any capital he could raise in some 'sure' American stock. A recession followed, and my father's scrapings of the barrel were lost. Lavington was heavily mortgaged and much of my mother's money was spent in an effort to keep it going; the cream of my grandfather's collection of books as well as valuable old furniture were sold. Mrs Winkworth, with a son and daughter, rented Lavington House for three summers at 25 guineas a week for six weeks and during this time we all moved to Beechwood. Her son Stephen fell in love with my eldest sister Dorothy (Dolly) who was eighteen, and they were married in 1895. I was one of eight bridesmaids and my pride in the bouquet of lilies-of-the-valley and the lovely brooch from the bridegroom was tremendous.

In 1904, after many legal negotiations and conferences, Lavington was sold to Mr James Buchanan of Black and White Whisky fame. In the general hubbub of sorting books and furniture to be stored I was allowed to sell the damsons from Beechwood. It was a bumper crop that year, and I kept the proceeds. This was a real windfall. A small furnished house was rented at Littlehampton as it was convenient for my father's County Council work and, possibly quite as important, there was an excellent golf course. I, meanwhile, was able to fish happily off the end of the pier. My mother, then fifty-six, had felt the wrench of leaving Lavington and had borne the brunt of all the organisation of the move from the only home she had known since marriage. She had a breakdown and went to my sister Dolly in London, where she was put to bed and made to rest.

And then, out of the blue, came disaster for me. Miss Lucy Phillimore, my mother's greatest friend, who always came to the rescue at any time of emergency, arrived to stay, and strongly disapproved of my spending my time fishing. I was sixteen years old, must really have some education, and was bundled off to St Hilda's School as a day girl. And I must be confirmed. It was no use arguing, so I bowed to the inevitable; after all, it might prove exciting. I was put in a class of girls of similar age and on the very first day in a thoroughly encouraging way the mistress in the Scripture lesson said, 'Well, you Octavia, as niece of the Bishop of Chichester, will know the answer to this question.' I blushed, felt it a bit below the belt to have relationships brought in and did *not* know the answer. Next, 'Don't slouch like a jellyfish.' I blushed again and for the first time in my life felt deeply hurt at the public insult. I stayed to the midday dinner and was given pork with sage and onion stuffing. I left it and was severely reprimanded for my lack of manners. I was introduced to Arithmetic, and moved into a class of little girls who were all superior to me in this horrible subject. I did know something about History and English, and at Dictation and Composition I generally came out top. My class mates seemed to have read nothing except Dickens, whose books I loathed. It was not till we played hockey that I gained even a modicum of respect from my school associates. Then my good eye and love of games served me well and I held my own.

I suffered agonies at the Confirmation class, though I knew it was a necessary step towards 'coming out'. At the end of the last class the Vicar spoke to each girl privately, and at the end of my interview he blessed me and kissed me warmly. He had a beard and I nearly hit him I was so outraged and shamed. Under vow of secrecy I confided in the one girl friend I had so far made, but she took it quite calmly and, as she was the daughter of a neighbouring parson, I wondered whether it was perhaps the accepted custom. I asked no other girl but I did complain to my family, who were satisfactorily indignant. Uncle Ernest, Bishop of Chichester, came to lunch before the Confirmation service; contrary to my fear that he might question me on the catechism and find me wanting, he paid no attention to me whatsoever, but discussed all the latest county gossip with my father. I was dressed afterwards in a white frock and behaved imperturbably. After all I was the Bishop's niece and next day I swaggered about his lunching with us.

After little more than a year in furnished houses in Little-hampton, Arundel and Rustington, when I used to bicycle daily to school at St Hilda's, my family found an unfurnished house large enough to take the furniture and pictures, at Bramlands, Henfield. With the move and settling in, I again drifted into an undisciplined manner of life. My only lessons were with Miss Margaret Macnamara who wrote plays, had a strong sense of humour, and was an authority on English Literature. I used to bicycle over to her house, Shiproda, where she taught me about Shakespeare.

Our first callers from the various neighbours in that part of Sussex were the Campions, who lived at Danny, a friendly Sussex atmosphere where there was talk of yesterday's hunt, golf at Pyecombe, and they were mad about games, like my family. I quickly struck up a friendship with Joan, the youngest child, who was a few years older than I was. She was an ideal friend for me, for she was always equable and cheerful. She was tall with large saxe-blue eyes and played the piano beautifully. Joan's other main occupations were hunting and making butter. I would sit happily reading my Shakespeare in the great hall with its mullioned windows and the heavenly smell from the large wood fire with its heap of white ashes against the old fireback. It was in this same hall that, in 1918, David Lloyd George drafted the terms of the Peace Treaty of the First World War. I was asked for weekends, shooting parties, tennis, golf, and met many cousins whose good manners and good looks often reduced me to bouts of shyness and a sense of conversational inadequacy.

Mrs Campion, who was said to be alarming because she was outspoken and blunt, was a rare personality. She was a shining example of practical voluntary service which achieved big results not hampered by her large, happy family of six children. She had started the Sunshine Home at Hurstpierpoint for convalescents, the Barclay Home for the Blind, Chichester House, a laundry in Hurstpierpoint for training workhouse girls, and was a pillar of the Mother's Union and I don't know how many other institutions. Her face was full of character and she would look at you with a twinkle in her eye. Shy and tongue-tied as I was, she put me at my ease and I was never afraid of her. She must have realised early how much I appreciated her and she told me, years later, that she always looked upon me as a fourth daughter. I felt at home with the Campions at Danny.

The Sydney Buxtons lived at Newtimber and it was Mrs Campion who said it would be nice for Phyllis Buxton to know me as we were the same age. Phyllis was a delicate girl and spent much of her time in a hut on the shoulder of Wolstonbury. She was a great reader and was the stepdaughter of the second Mrs Buxton. Phyllis and I soon became friends and I found her blunt, tactless, reserved and with a heart of gold. She seemed to care as much as I did for poetry and had read more. I taught her to play golf at Pyecombe and she was very keen but, unlike Joan, she had not been brought up on games. My time became largely divided between Joan at Danny and Phyllis at Pyecombe.

[The Liberal Buxtons were in marked contrast to the Conservative Campions.] I was invited to Newtimber and 'looked over' by the vigilant eyes of Mrs Buxton and the possessive governess Miss Mitchell. The Buxtons were essentially studious, and I was a little overawed by the political, intellectual atmosphere. Sydney Buxton was Postmaster-General [in the Liberal Cabinet] and I was a little afraid of him. He was always busy with Cabinet papers, fussing over plans and calling for his daughter or his wife. He and his wife were constantly away and, being Liberals, were not at first much welcomed in Sussex social circles. I was happier with Phyllis on the Downs at Pyecombe than at Newtimber.

There was also a big contrast between Mrs Campion and Mrs Buxton. The Postmaster-General's wife at Newtimber struck me as a hard-working, subservient, conscientious wife. She was constantly involved in social and political activities on behalf of the Liberals and her husband's Poplar constituency. Her husband always came first and I used to feel annoyed when, after arranging for golf at Pyecombe on Saturday, Phyllis would ring up and say, 'Daddy has come back earlier and he may want me so I can't play today.' But Mrs Buxton was full of common sense, adored her children and her garden. No one could have been a better stepmother to Charlie and Phyllis and it was never obvious that 'Mum', as they affectionately called her, was not their real mother. Her own twins, Denis and Doreen, were much younger than Phyllis, and a most original couple. Charlie, Phyllis's brother, the only surviving son of the first Mrs Buxton, was tall, wore spectacles and shared his father's enthusiasm for fishing. He wrote poetry and was constantly reciting it. He was devoted to Phyllis and Doreen and guided Phyllis in her choice of books. His political views were a source of much anxiety to his father for he was very left wing, and had a profound faith in the future of labour.

In the summer of 1908 the Buxtons invited me to Skeabost in the Isle of Skye. There was a large party of cousins and I enjoyed it all enormously. I got to know Phyllis much better and we would go for long expeditions, sightseeing, deer stalking or fishing with Charlie. There was much feeble-minded, hilarious ragging, and salmon to eat so often that even I became tired of it! I was rather attracted by Charlie's gentleness and by the Buxton standards of general domestic comfort. But from the point of view of possible marriage, I found the Campion's young men friends, games-loving and fond of shooting and parties, more my intellectual level and easier to get on with.

My mother began to be resentful of my outside interests and my preoccupation with Danny. When I returned from there, or if I chanced to be delayed, I came to realise I would meet with black disapproval. It worried me. My mother had taken advice as to how to make the most of the available lawn at Bramlands for roses. Beds were cut out of the turf and I took charge of the planting, and pruned and cherished the many selections of roses. I joined the National Rose Society. I studied all the literature and taught myself everything I could; the roses, loving the heavy virgin clay soil, responded and made a fine show.

I was also useful over the housekeeping, and it was arranged that I should stay with my mother's sister, Aunt Betty Milbanke, in London, where I took a course at the Buckingham Palace Road School of Cookery. I enjoyed this and loved Aunt Betty, but I got a bad attack of laryngitis which alarmed her and her doctor, and as soon as I was better I was sent home. Evidently that sort of life was dangerous for a girl with a weak throat! I am now disposed to view the 'weak throat' as a convenient excuse for keeping me at home! Certainly my affection for dear Aunt Betty was resented.

My brother John had always been my mother's favourite. He became desperately ill with a high temperature which was at first thought to be influenza but was finally diagnosed as typhoid fever. I had a difficult time trying to keep my mother from collapsing with anxiety and the two nurses from being bored. It was a terribly anxious time and John had several relapses. One of the nurses became a great friend of mine. In her off-duty time I would take her for walks and she would talk about her past cases by the hour. She encouraged me to get out of the house and to play golf and was an exceptionally kind person. She was the one and only individual who could manage John whether in the delirium of fever or the tedious weariness of his convalescence.

About this time [1907–8] it was decided that I should be presented at Court. Miss Lucy Phillimore, [my mother's friend], undertook to pay for my outfit and I had to go to London for fittings. Even I, with no flair for clothes, was impressed by the grandeur of the white satin gown and the rose patterned damask silk of my train. I looked altogether unrecognisable in my Court dress with ostrich feathers on my head. I had to practise the curtsey and an upright posture. We had the entrée through the good offices of my mother's nephew, Lord Denman, who was a Lord-in-Waiting. This, a little, speeded up the brougham in its slow progress along the Mall – a great relief for me as I was prone to carriage sickness. [Inside Buckingham Palace] we were ushered along, lined up, and our names duly called. I managed my curtsey without mishap to the much-medalled, magnificently uniformed King Edward VII. He had the appearance of being interested in each presentation, while the beautiful, but rigid Queen Alexandra kept her eyes on the ceiling. Did the unending stream that bobbed up and down in front of her make her feel seasick? It must have been a boring trial of endurance. We were lucky to have good positions afterwards and could watch the other presentations and particularly the expressions of the Court in attendance behind Their Majesties.

I was now officially out and better still had two really good frocks for the few dances I went to, invitations for which were usually due to my sister Dolly. I was definitely flattered when a young Irish officer asked to be introduced to me rather than my prettier sisters. He was a beautiful dancer and made me eat mangoes at supper and drink champagne. When we parted, the attractive Irishman asked if I was going next night to a certain ball and we were both disappointed that I was not. I could easily have lost my heart to his cheerful, graceful manner and his attractively crooked mouth. At another dance a young doctor tried to kiss me and, as I'd never seen him before, I was profoundly shocked. 'But don't you like it?' he asked with apparent surprise. I decided he was plainly bad form.

After a brief taste of London life I returned to my rose growing, my Sussex friends and my golf. I won several competitions at Pyecombe and a Challenge Rose Bowl at the Southdown Golf Club at Shoreham. The first time I won it was in 1907, I lost it in 1908 and 1909, but in 1910 swept the board and won it with other prizes and a good bit of money. It had not been very difficult, I came to the conclusion, one only had to keep one's eye on the ball and concentrate with grim determination. Though my golf success helped my self-confidence it was, after all, only a game and at intervals I felt depressed. I confided this to Phyllis and found that she too had her moments of depression due largely to her not being the social success that her stepmother expected. I could not see that it really greatly mattered, that if she wanted to get married and have a dozen children she probably would when the right man came along.

Mine was a deeper depression. I had no desire to tread in my sisters' footsteps. I wanted something else, though I was ready to fall in love if an ideal young man came along. I knew I was ambitious and would like to write. I adored poetry and wrote verses to Joan and the Sussex Downs, but knew I could never be a first-class poet. I did the housekeeping for the family but, apart from rose growing, most of my energies were devoted to games. Mixed hockey occupied a good deal of time in the winter, and tennis and sometimes cricket or stoolball in the summer. I would like to mean something in the world. But how?

2

THE TURNING POINT
Marriage or Education?
1909–11

In the early summer of 1909, [when I was twenty-one,] I met Elizabeth Robins. It was a turning point in my life. She was an American actress who had toured the US with Edwin Booth and had come over in 1888 on a supposedly short visit to Norway and England, but had succumbed to the magnetism of this country and had made it her home. She had plunged gaily into London society and, with the help of many of the leading literary figures of the day, including Oscar Wilde, Henry James, George Bernard Shaw and William Archer, had made her way on the London stage. At that time she was particularly interested in Ibsen, and was largely responsible for introducing his plays to London, making a lasting impression in the parts of Hedda Gabler and, above all, of Hilde in *The Master Builder*. Her last appearance on the stage was in *Paola and Francesca* in 1908 but she had already settled down to making her living by writing. The publication of *The Open Question* in 1898, under the pseudonym of C.E. Raimond, had created a literary sensation, though the betrayal of her identity by Mrs Patrick Campbell discouraged her from writing for a time. Phyllis told me something about her reputation as a best-seller and said that I should read *The Magnetic North*, first published in 1904, which was about Alaska. She had read it on the hottest summer day in a hayfield and it had made her shiver.

I had always read omnivorously and longed to write myself, and to meet so distinguished an author in the flesh was a terrific adventure. It was a small family luncheon at Newtimber and Elizabeth Robins was dressed in a blue suit, the colour of speedwell, which matched her beautiful deep-set eyes. I was introduced as Phyllis's friend who lived near Henfield. 'A neighbour then?' said Elizabeth Robins, and with a charming grace and in an unforgettable voice asked me if I would come to tea one day and she would show me her modest little garden. I palpitatingly said 'I'd love to', and she paid not a moment's further attention to me. The conversation was about gardens, personalities in the Liberal party and the latest books. Elizabeth Robins was an enthralling and witty talker.

For several days after this nothing happened, and then came a brief note asking me to come to tea. I went, and was very impressed by the book-lined walls and the photographs of literary celebrities. I was asked if I knew Henley's poems, and Stevenson's *The Lantern Bearers*? I falteringly answered, 'no'. Then I must come one day and she would read them to me if I liked. I said I'd love to. 'But what is the matter with this rose? Mildred says you know so much about rose growing and do all the pruning at Bramlands where they are a wonderful show.' I tried to pose as an expert since I belonged to the National Rose Society and read all their books. I advised syringing with quassia and soft soap solution. 'May I come and do that for you? I'll bring my own syringe.' Perhaps if I could make myself useful in this way I might one day get some advice on how to write myself. It was a case of hero-worship at first sight.

I syringed her roses until there could not have been one greenfly left in Henfield village and helped to weed out the Devil's Guts (ground elder) in her garden. I bicycled over at 6 a.m. and watered the garden until she looked out of her window and saw me there. She became aware of me and a little interested and asked me what I wanted to do with my life besides grow roses and play golf. 'Write,' I said, diffidently and desperately. 'But my dear, you can't write until you have lived and have known a great deal more about life,' she said with conviction. I felt crushed, but the blow was softened by the kindness in her voice.

Soon after this she went up north to Rounton to stay with the Hugh Bells and I was allowed to look in on the garden and write to tell her how things were getting on. Florence, Lady

Bell, stepmother of Gertrude Bell and wife of Sir Hugh Bell, the ironmaster, was her closest, dearest friend – her 'blest companion' from the earliest Ibsen days. As early as 1897 she had written a comedy *L'Indécis*, and was invariably to be found in the front row on London first nights. Miss Robins visited Rounton several times a year when she was stale and tired from too many London activities; she never failed to be revived, and her writing inspired, by the stimulating friendship and the bracing Yorkshire air. They corresponded regularly, always weekly, and not infrequently daily. I felt that Lady Bell must be an exceptional woman; for though she strongly disapproved of the agitation for Women's Suffrage which Miss Robins ardently supported, it made no difference to their close friendship.

When Miss Robins came back from the North my mother called on her. My family was curious about this intriguing newcomer to Henfield, this authoress imported by the Buxtons, who was said to be a Suffragette, a friend of H.G. Wells and of George Moore – neither of them of very savoury reputation as regards women. Miss Robins asked my parents to tea and, as my mother was away from home, I was sent to chaperone my impressionable father. She said how much she admired my godfather, Uncle Basil, and his wife was at once written to for credentials. Aunt Charlotte replied, 'Elizabeth Robins streaks across the London sky from time to time like a meteor.' My shopping expeditions to Henfield became more frequent and took longer and I was questioned about this. I drove Miss Robins about the countryside in the dogcart and showed her views from the Downs, and lent her volumes of the Sussex Archaeological Society. I was greatly impressed at the range of my new friend's knowledge. I often popped into Backset to water a special rose bush, hoping to catch a glimpse of Elizabeth Robins. But remembering my family's antagonism to my friendship with Joan Campion, I was secretive and invented excuses for my prolonged absences.

Both Joan Campion and I were afflicted by a sense of our abysmal ignorance. My education had been as brief as a butterfly's flight on a summer's day. Joan, brought up by governesses, knew more, but when we listened to the conversations between the Buxtons and Miss Robins about every subject under the sun, and literature in particular, we felt sadly out of our depth. We took a bold step and consulted both Mrs Campion and Miss Robins as to how we might improve our education. We firmly said that our families must not know or we should be mocked and life would be insupportable, and that only these two must share our discreditable secret. They both thought it a praiseworthy idea, and Miss Robins wrote to consult Miss Penelope Lawrence, Headmistress of Roedean. The answer came that her staff did not normally take on outside work but she had a brilliant young woman who taught the sixth form, a Miss Sybil Wragge, who might be willing to help us. This was encouraging news and we at once began to make plans. We plainly could not use our own names and should have to pretend to be playing golf while making our visit to Roedean. It was decided that I should take the tandem bicycle up to Pyecombe golf course and meet Joan there, taking sandwiches for lunch while we played, not golf, but truant. It was a warm day in late May. As we pedalled along, we were sweating with apprehension as well as heat as we saw the imposing Roedean buildings before us. I wrote a description of our adventure to Miss Robins for her approval:

Well! we got to Roedean, a huge place on a cliff three miles to the East of Brighton, overlooking the sea. We asked for Miss Wragge and remembered with a shock that our names were Denny! The great Miss Wragge was quite young, 23 to 28, with brown intelligent probing eyes that were intensely puzzled by us!! No wonder, poor thing. We said we wanted to know something about poets and men of letters of 18th or 19th century as we knew nothing much about them. She suggested we should begin with Wordsworth and Coleridge as they started a new lot of poets and she was very much interested in them herself. Then she said 'But why have you suddenly decided to do this, what made you?' We explained we found ourselves so ignorant and we thought it would be a good thing to learn a little. She was much mystified. I didn't say I had been stirred up by your 'impassioned eloquence'.

She asked what we expected her to do. Did we want her to place Wordsworth in his position in the history of literature for us? She was most anxious to know our ideas and most willing to oblige. Joan suggested I should ask Miss Robins. She said 'I have been wondering; is this Miss Elizabeth Robins the great writer?' We said 'Yes'. More and greater amazement on her part. I'm sure she thought, 'What *can* Miss Robins have thought about these two rather unintelligent, ignorant girls.' She little knew it was only just pure kindness on your part. However, I shan't tell her that, she is very much interested in us, and she must remain so, until she finds us out! Meanwhile next Friday we are to go and every Friday until 2 July when Joan goes to Homburg with her parents. It's an awfully short time, just long enough to get thoroughly interested in a thing and then – well! Joan says I am not to go without her.

We asked Miss Wragge what we should pay her, an embarrassing question, and I think it was 7/6d a time. She looked at us with considerable surprise when we said we had come twelve or thirteen miles on a tandem bicycle because it saved fares. (I subsisted on about £1 a month and my mother paid for my clothes and fares. A godmother had luckily left me £100 so that I felt uncommonly rich at that moment, and could pay tuition fees.) We then gave her our real names and explained about letters. I asked that mine should be sent to Backset as my family always opened and read my letters, and she accepted the situation as a joke but laughingly said, 'Surely nobody would tease you over wanting to learn?' But in those days brothers only wanted a social success and a rich brother-in-law for their sisters.

We both found that Miss Wragge had high standards and was very particular about the meaning of words and the English we wrote. Joan was then twenty-five and it was late to begin so that we must have seemed an odd pair, but I hope we were a refreshing experience by contrast with the well-trained sixth-form brains of Roedean. At least we did our best. We worked hard at Wordsworth and Miss Wragge promoted us to Carlyle, Coleridge and Shelley. I found it most exciting trying to get inside Wordsworth's mind but Joan began to get bored with learning.

In January 1911 Miss Robins went to a spa in Germany for her health and I missed her greatly 'as a windmill must feel when the wind doesn't blow'. In a letter to her I said:

I've been attending to my rose cuttings which are planted in sand, light, gritty stuff, and they remain quite healthy so long as their roots don't go deeper into the heavier, stronger soil beneath the sand. They mustn't do that until the sun is warmer. In some ways the same treatment is required for me, for until Backset became such a large feature in my life I was a sort of cutting with sand at my feet, and poor stuff it was too. Well then luckily I was rescued from that wretched sand and my roots were put into a backsettian soil made of really good sound stuff. Look how well your roses do! And the educational variety of roots you planted in Shelley, Stevenson, Shakespeare, etc., with Wragge as under-gardener. But then, besides that brand there is another more personal lot of roots from the very heart of the plant, and they go very deep and, owing to your gentle, tender care, would not be pulled up. They can't grow now as you are away and the soil is hard and frozen. The roses are covered with dead leaves.

I wrote screeds about the Downs and their superiority to people, especially Society with a large S. I was adolescent and inexperienced with all the intolerance of youth, with a thirst for beauty, with romantic ideals, but observant in everyday life and not devoid of humour or Miss Robins might rapidly have tired of my letters.

I stayed a weekend at Danny and wrote to her:

I bicycled to see Joan. She is on the same level in the family's eyes as you were before you went abroad and, in a silent way, objects are placed to prevent, or make it harder, for me to go there. But nothing is said because I seize every opportunity of singing praises of the Campions with a touch of defiance that makes it more amusing to me to watch the effect. It seems people must be given absurd things to think about or they look for trouble where there is none.

My family [went away for a fortnight] in March as the house had to be spring cleaned and all the maids were to be away; but I could stay and be looked after by Edith Elliott, the gardener's wife. I was passionately anxious for this plan to come off as then I could enjoy working at Miss Wragge's stuff, really concentrating; if Miss Robins returned we could have afternoons on the Downs and more readings of poetry – or prose.

Miss Robins's return was postponed, so I continued to write to her my views of life. 'When I knew you hardly at all, I unconsciously took great trouble to be truthful to you in all I said. And I always wanted to treat you with perfect frankness.' I was then twenty-three years old and most happy playing games, growing roses, making visits, going to occasional dances. But there was another side of me which became depressed at the laziness of my character, my lack of education, the uselessness of my life. I worked off emotion in hero-worship and my love of my native Sussex and the Downs. I tried to put my feelings into verse. Although I disapproved of the way my sisters flirted I had my own romantic ideas and I might have fallen in love and married an ideal young man. I paid a visit to Dorothy Pleydell Bouverie, a gifted musician who adored my mother. She talked to me for three hours on my first night. 'Have you ever been in love,' she said, 'it would soften you.' But she added, 'I'd be sorry for the man who married you. You're too critical.' This was a new aspect of myself, and I was mildly amused, for I had never been seriously in love.

[In a series of long letters, Octavia described to Elizabeth Robins the personal crisis caused by Charles Buxton's proposal.

An odd talk with the Buxton's governess, Miss Mitchell, a year before the proposal, should have prepared Octavia:]

Last year when I had the misfortune to sprain my ankle, staying with the Buxtons in Scotland, I couldn't do anything for a day or two but stay indoors on a sofa. They all went out and left me, I remember, one particular day, all except Miss Mitchell. She wouldn't go. She didn't stop talking and she bored me nearly to death. At last she discussed the Buxton family, and for every virtue that it is possible for mortals to possess, according to Miss Mitchell, the rest of the world hasn't a chance. Then she asked me if I didn't agree. I said she knew them better than I did, and probably she was right; anyhow I thought them all very nice. Upon that, she was kind enough to suggest that I should marry Charlie Buxton! I was so amused that I laughed till I ached. That rather offended her and she asked me what I meant and said he was so handsome. I tried to explain that I thought it rather an odd conversation and that at that moment I was not, strange as it might seem to her, contemplating marrying anybody. She wouldn't believe this extraordinary – as it seemed to her – statement. Did I like him? I said he seemed quite nice, but even that I said doubtfully! It amused me to think that that huge lanky boy should be championed in this valiant way by that very small creature. As for the rest I've played golf with him and Phyllis, and found him harmless but uninteresting.

[But in March 1911 Octavia could no longer evade the unpleasant experience of an unwelcome proposal of marriage, as she explained to Miss Robins:]

[On Saturday 11 March I get down late for breakfast after a night in London.] My mother hovers in and out of my bedroom while I'm dressing. At breakfast I get this letter:

Dear Miss Tate,
    Phyllis tells me you are going to Bramlands tomorrow. I shall walk over from Newtimber after luncheon, reaching

Bramlands at about 2.15, as I want particularly to speak
to you.
Yours very sincerely,
Charles S. Buxton

I am surprised and much annoyed. I go up to my mother
and begin talking about ordinary things. Suddenly she says:
'You've heard from Charlie Buxton this morning.'

I say 'Yes, but how *did* you know that?'

Then she begins, 'I didn't mean to tell you, but Thursday
night a messenger boy arrived with a note from Mrs Buxton
saying, "I must see you on a matter of great importance,
shall I come and see you or will you come here?"' My mother
arranged to go there. Thank heavens Dolly wasn't in when
the boy arrived or the whole family would know of the
business already. She went to Buckingham Gate Friday afternoon. (All the time she is telling the story I make frivolous
remarks with a smile that stiffens painfully as I realise what
an infernal nuisance it's all going to be.) Mrs Buxton makes
a piteous, moving tale to the effect that Charlie has been so
badly in love with me that it's a wonder he hasn't faded quite
away, since I stayed with them in Skye three years ago. And
then a lot of silly rot such as my being one in a thousand
and Charlie was too – Why do people make such absurdly
ridiculous remarks? Would my mother be against it and had
Tate ever said anything about him. No, my mother wasn't
against him and the connection would be so delightful and
all the usual conventional remarks. She also adds Tate had
never said anything about him at all. The last three weeks he
had been miserable wanting to speak, all the time, and generally making himself a nuisance to the rest of his family. All
the Buxtons are so fond of me and would like it so much.
Finally my mother says she won't mention it to me and lets
out (damn it all) that I'm alone here [at Bramlands] and since
he's in such a hurry he had better get it over. I make many
meant-to-be amusing remarks during it all and finally with a
quick lapse into seriousness say, 'I'm most awfully sorry but
I don't approve of marrying people one doesn't particularly

like, do you?' She agrees but says I must be kind to him. I ask her how many people in my family know of it – only John who had advised her to treat it lightly and leave it to me. She says I'll have to get over it some time and the sooner the better. I swear internally.

I arrive home in rain. I arrange [by letter] 3 p.m. for Charlie Buxton. I'm still terribly miserable at the thought of an ordeal like this. I eat a nondescript meal.

Sunday. I arrange to send the cart for my singing mistress (Fannie Wood), who has been ill, to bring her to tea at 4 today. Somebody had to be collected or how am I to get rid of that boy, when I want?

I come to the conclusion that it's the duty of mothers to insist on girls doing things for *their own* happiness and pleasure and not from a sense of duty, or because by doing things they please other people. I am thankful firstly to Joan because she first encouraged me to be selfish and do things to please myself and not other people. John's nurse did too. And finally *you*. Four, three or two years ago if this had happened I should have thought, 'Oh well it seems it will make him very happy. I may as well marry Charlie Buxton, I like him all right.' Result? Who can tell? It might have been all right or it might not.

3.20. He came and we went for a walk along the lane, making careful conversation about everyday affairs.

Then: 'Tate, is it any good, do you think you could care for me?'

'I'm so dreadfully sorry. I wish you wouldn't go on. I'm afraid I don't.' I feel I would walk into hell with alacrity to avoid this interview.

'Don't you think you ever could? It would help me so much and I'm sure,' with rather a defiant jerk of his head in a proud way, 'I'm sure you could make something of me.'

I prod holes in the mud with my stick, not knowing what words would be least brutal.

Then I say, 'I've always liked you and looked on you as just a relation of Phyllis'; not much point in that remark but

I'm quite as miserable as he is. He wore no hat, red bow tie, and primroses in his button hole.

'Is it any good my trying again?'

Involuntarily I cry beseechingly 'Oh! not again soon.'

He, very gravely, 'No not soon.'

Again I say, 'I'm dreadfully sorry but I really don't care, and I can't help it, can I?'

With a ghastly smile he says, 'Well, will you shake hands?'

'Oh yes,' *very* relieved that it really has come to an end! Then solemnly we shake hands and two miserably wretched eyes through spectacles burn themselves on to my brain in a way I shan't forget quickly. We say 'Goodbye' and I return along that lane, covered with twigs and leaves and hard flints, my head bowed and viciously hitting every leaf I can with my stick.

I write to my mother and say that the boy has gone, ending with, 'I'm so awfully sorry he should be so miserable. I am not like the rest of your daughters who have a readiness to fall in love with great rapidity!'

A few days later I received a wire from Miss Robins in Germany saying, 'Good girl', which cheered me and I burned a joss stick in celebration, as I felt I had her thoughts to comfort me.

There was no doubt that my family considered Charlie Buxton as a most eligible *parti*, a nice person, and that I should be happily off their hands and well provided for as soon as I was married to him. They questioned me closely as to what had happened between us, and why I had refused to marry him. Whenever I was alone, trying to study, my mother would tackle me and, with a frantic desire to escape, I went more and more frequently to Backset and, when I was sure Charlie wasn't there, to Newtimber. On my return from one of these Backset outings I wrote to Miss Robins:

I was amazed when I got in to hear all the old worn out things about women's friendships, and what had I been doing with you. 'Chattering?' – with the utmost scorn. It seems you said not very complimentary things about men in *The*

Dark Lantern and it is apparently feared you might run them
down to my young and guiltless mind, or even go so far as
to encourage me not to marry. I said you are very careful
what you say and it was all great nonsense and the same old
story that any friend I made was bound to be run-down. I
also said 'Of course she is a Suffragette and doubtless thinks,
as they all do, that she is equal to men.' Really, the things
they think they can say to me. 'Had you a nice mind?' I was
asked. I was calm and wearily patient and deigned to explain
you had never in your life shocked me.

They are fools, John and my mother. I'm such an easy
person to get on with if I'm not interfered with, while I
might be the very devil if they expect me to be tied to them
with a chain. After all, old William [Wilberforce] moved
heaven and earth to free those slaves. Suppose I inherited
equal energy in freeing myself? If there *is* anything in
heredity. I want so little, and if there is trouble it will be
their fault.

During this 'female friendship' barrage, examples were
quoted of the devotion of sisters to brothers in fiction, and
my mother said, 'Of course Shakespeare never depicted female
friends.' I sat quiet, always ready to escape an argument if there
were several opponents. I felt I wasn't clever enough to keep
my end up against more than one at a time. But to my amazement Susan said, 'Oh well, what about Rosalind and Celia,
Helena and Hermia, Portia and Nerissa?' I appeared bored and
indifferent, curled up on the sofa, but deep inside I chuckled
to myself with glee!

By degrees I began to gain courage, largely because Miss
Robins had told me that 'I must fight against being afraid'.
Neither she nor Joan realised what it was like to be so afraid,
the weariness of coming to the surface to breathe, only to have
something fresh aimed at one. But that mood was becoming
rarer and I was beginning to feel a certain stimulation in having
so many hands raised against me. But one evening in a mood
of despair I wrote to Miss Robins:

It is probably imagination but I've somehow felt that you have been treating me very carefully since your return, [perhaps] because you think I ought to marry that boy. If one never bothers about any selfish happiness but just trots along on the surface of things, then one avoids – well the mood I'm in tonight. Instead of getting down a bit deeper into life and caring about things with a good deal of seriousness, I almost think it better to swing right back and care *nothing*, in the acting-a-part sort of existence I led at one time. And that you know is heresy.

I was upbraided for weakness, and apologised, a few days later.

At about this time the nurse who had looked after John during his illness came to stay for a short holiday and a rest from her hospital work. She discovered the reason for my looking ill and depressed and sensed the tension I was under, and the atmosphere of nagging coercion which surrounded me. She urged me to get away as much as possible. I had refused an invitation to go away, and my mother was displeased: 'I like you to go about and see people while you are *still young*,' she had said with biting emphasis. I was bitterly disappointed when a yachting expedition with the Rendels had to be cancelled as I had hoped for time to think things out, away from the restrictions and the mesmeric tyranny of Bramlands. My every movement was watched and if I wanted to write a letter to Miss Robins pouring out my feelings, it had to be written in the bath behind the locked door.

As a consequence I took every opportunity to be left alone. My main object was peace at any price, and I cared little what deceits I used to attain my aim. There came a day when I was deep in some gardening operation at Backset when a sister turned up – she had been sent to find me and take me home. 'You've been here hours,' she said accusingly in front of Miss Robins. I was taken away in disgrace and told I was not to go there so often. I was furious and went, as soon as possible, to complain to Miss Robins about the restrictions which had been imposed on me. Instead of meeting with the expected sympathy I was bewildered to find myself attacked by my friend who had

had no idea that I was concealing my visits to her. She was very angry indeed. 'Straightness and truth are essential foundations to all that is best in life,' she said. I felt a deceitful worm and apologised and she seemed slightly mollified. She made me promise that, if our friendship was to go on, it must be on a basis of truth and openness. But how was I to see as much of her as I wanted if I had to tell my family each time? I had already learned my lesson by bitter experience over the Campions. Truth was something nobody had ever talked to me about – what terribly high standards this woman had – she who was supposed to be hardly fit to know! I went home and tried to find comfort in Bacon's essays on 'Truth' and 'Friendship'. Life seemed unbearable and, besides, Phyllis and Joan were both away so that I had nobody even to get away and play golf with.

On 9 June I had another letter from Charlie. By the grace of God I met the postman so that my family knew nothing about it. He returned to the charge and asked me if there was still no hope. I spent hours that night trying to write a firm but not unkind reply and finally sent it to Miss Robins to read and send on if she felt I had adequately covered the ground.

The constant harrowing at home was having the effect of turning me in upon myself, making my roots go deeper, helping me to grow up. I was constantly subjected to remarks on why did I not wish to marry Charlie Buxton. It became unbearable and got on my nerves. I lost weight – largely through being unable to eat my meals without fear of arguments. I worked myself up to a frantic degree in an outburst to Miss Robins in the following letter:

9 June 1911

When I was eighteen I would have married anything that might have asked me if I thought it would have been advantageous and conducive to fun. Didn't believe in any silly rot like love and I might have been the most amenable daughter alive. From that time onwards I never thought about the matter from a *personal* point of view.

When that letter came in London I was most awfully sorry

and wished I had never seen the boy. I was perfectly miserable and from trying to imagine how he felt I almost felt I was a criminal. I didn't think about myself at all except in a dull way I knew it was utterly impossible. When he came and I walked along the lane with him I felt I was a beast and quite dreadfully sorry. But when he spoke of it, though he *said* quite nice things, I suddenly felt so revolted at what it all meant from *my* point of view. I was so staggered at the horror of such thoughts that (I didn't tell you this before) to prevent the sleeve of his coat touching mine I walked in the ditch! If I have ever grown up it was at that moment. Anyhow I suddenly saw a great many things horribly realistically and it completely took my breath away. And among other things I felt I was on the same level as an animal.

But if he had gone on to say any more than he did I could have picked up the stones from the road and hurled them at him. As it was I pulled myself together, tried to summon some of the sorryness I had felt before for him, but which had suddenly died and shrunk to nothing, and I behaved fairly decently. But I was really absolutely dazed and felt I had come up against something too horrible for words and which I could not understand. And that awful look. Ugh! The sort of greedy way a particularly greedy old mutual acquaintance eyes the strawberry dish, a craving for possession. No, I'm not going to think about that any more or it will get on my nerves again. Only I did want you to understand a little. Well, after a little while I covered up and tried to ignore the fact that I had ever opened my eyes for a moment. Sometimes I was successful, sometimes not. What simply dug itself into my mind was the beauty of friendship. When I could think of that, and of you, I was a little consoled.

Some people are cut out for marriage; they are made for it and would be most happy in it. Perhaps people are made differently, but I am *not* cut out for it. Everybody I know would be shocked and horrified at that statement and at this: the very thought of it makes me shudder and it revolts me. This will not be said to anyone else if I retain my senses.

Methinks if I ever get married I should have to be frantically and disgustingly in love. As for money, I would become a lady golf-professional or a sweaty cook rather than . . . the other. These are the thoughts I have managed to conceal from you – and perhaps after all you knew them – since you came back from abroad and everybody in turn failed me. The world is made in a beastly way too. I am fond of Mrs Buxton in a way and she used to be very kind to me. Why? Only because she hoped to have me as a daughter-in-law, Phyllis owned that. And now in that family I am a beast and a criminal, and in this, merely an awful young fool.

In Victorian times I should probably have been ripe for a 'decline'; in these days I should have been given psychiatric treatment. Instead I had to battle through by my own resources combined with valiant bolstering up from Joan and wonderful understanding friendship from Phyllis.

My family's relentless campaign to force me into marriage undoubtedly hardened my determination to possess my own spirit – never to be a slave! In my formative years sex was never discussed, but as the youngest of a large family with knowledge gained from a country upbringing and an inquisitive mind I was not wholly ignorant of its power, nor of what was then accepted as its purpose. I believed that, however pleasurable and exciting, its primary function was procreation. I was fully alive to the fact that some individuals – as some animals – were far more susceptible to sex attraction – domination even – than others. But this seemed to be only in line with other appetites, such as food or drink. However keen the urge, as I advanced in years I wanted more and more to keep free from being governed by my body.

*   *   *

[Three months later,] the heat was sweltering and the family were away. Mrs Rodgers came in from shopping at Hurstpierpoint, where she had heard that Charlie Buxton had been rushed home to Newtimber and been operated on for appendicitis. The following day, 31 August 1911, Phyllis sent me over a note to say that Charlie was dead. It was an appalling shock. I went over in my mind the visits to Scotland in previous years and realised how closely I had become woven into that family life and how I felt the sense of unity which existed between Charlie and Phyllis. We used to tease them and call them the Affinities. How would she get on without him? Large and awkward, he was always gentle and considerate to me; once when I grew homesick and bored with all the party, he was the only one who didn't really jar on me when he talked.

I consulted Miss Robins who said I must certainly write and offer to go over. I did this and Phyllis replied to my note, 'Do come'. She met me, her face white and grief-stricken, and took me upstairs; though I would have liked to refuse, I felt it was expected of me. His was the first dead body I had ever seen and I was left alone with him lying there surrounded by flowers, peaceful with all the majesty of death. It was an unforgettable experience. I was profoundly moved and made miserable by thinking of the unhappiness and disappointment I brought him. I remember his letter from Wye when he said, 'Give us a chance, as schoolboys say.' I wished I had been the least bit nice to him, and yet I was thankful in a sense that I was never induced to marry him since I didn't care for him in the right way and he was too good to be sacrificed to that sort of thing – a marriage for money, or for convenience.

Late that night I went out and gazed at the heavens and wished as I saw a-shooting star. It was clear and crisp, everything so much alive, and now and again a faint rustle in some tree disturbed the silence only known to the night.

3
'WHY COULDN'T *I* BECOME A DOCTOR?'
1911–12

Janet, our late housemaid, who married the postman, had a hacking cough. I was extremely worried about her and visited her constantly. I was much attached to Janet and she would talk very frankly to me about many aspects of life, her round olive green eyes looking directly at me from her high cheek bones and ruddy complexion. My intervention over her health absorbed a good deal of my care and consideration. There was no mass radiography and far less use of X-rays in 1911. Three or four doctors in surrounding villages had seen her at my request and they each assured me that her cough was nothing serious. It was magnified in her own mind by the fact that her mother had died of consumption. There they were wrong. Janet herself accepted the cough as more or less normal and thought I was being unduly fussy. She reminded me how well she had been while pregnant (a common happening as I soon afterwards learned.) Naturally it was worse and she had lost weight with the care she had to give to her beloved baby and it was tiresome of me when I insisted on her seeing a woman doctor, Dr Louisa Martindale in Brighton.

This time it was a longer examination and an X-ray of her chest, confirmed later by a sputum test, backed up the clinical diagnosis that only a part of one lung was not affected by tuberculosis. I was enraged by the delay in not catching the trouble at an earlier stage. I took her to Brompton Hospital. 'Too advanced for admission.' I boiled over with fury to Phyllis; after all, if I with only my eyes and no stethoscope had been able to diagnose tuberculosis all those months ago I could be a better doctor myself.

In a mood of complete despondency I grumbled to Miss Robins. In my abysmal ignorance of what a medical training involved, I told her that my observations and common sense had proved me right in diagnosis. 'Why couldn't *I* become qualified and be a doctor . . .' She turned and looked at me with flashing eyes and an expression I'd never seen in them before and burst out: 'Now that would be a worthwhile life. My father wanted me, urged me, to be a doctor,' and with passionate enthusiasm, 'It's the greatest profession in the world.'

I was flabbergasted! What had I started? After a moment I hesitantly began, 'I could certainly come to know people in the raw – no Society frills' . . . She took this up and dilated further on the opportunities and rewards for a first-class doctor. There was little doubt that I had suddenly earned a new respect from this wonderful friend. I talked to Joan and she too was full of valiant exhortation. My family was a sobering thought. I knew they'd always be against any plan that took me away from home except for a suitable marriage.

Soon after this Phyllis asked me if I'd seen much of Miss Robins lately. She reported that Miss Robins had had a long talk with her mother about me and said she was exceedingly fond of me. I was quite overwhelmed and asked what she had said about me, to which Phyllis said: 'Oh! she said you had a nice character and liked poetry.' She emphasised *how* lucky I was to have Miss Robins as a friend and 'Don't you feel you are her devoted slave for ever more?' 'Yes, indeed,' I replied.

The following day I went off to play golf for Sussex and was indoctrinated by the rest of the team as to how important a match it was. If we won we should tie with Surrey for the championship. I must not be nervous and they did their best to stir up loyalty for Sussex (hardly necessary in my case!). My loyalty to Sussex plus luck won me the match. I was taken on one side and hurriedly told I was not to say this was my first match playing for Sussex. I was congratulated by everybody as if it had been a matter of life and death. My mother was not pleased. She had heard that these golfing women were ravening wolves and corrupted the young. I learned that a friend of

Dolly's had said they smoked and drank and even called each other by their surnames! Aunt Betty redressed the balance, 'How splendid! I feel quite proud of you.'

I had plenty of time to think in a fresh atmosphere [during a visit to my cousin, Herbert W. Wilberforce, in Yorkshire]. I thought about my mother and realised how fond I was of her. She was a highly gifted, unique woman who treated me with sympathy and understanding, except for her fanatical obsession about my future. This I felt was partly due to my brother John's influence and partly to the fact that she was continually worried over money and how to make both ends meet. To get another daughter adequately provided for was a highly desirable aim. I had now made up my mind to study Medicine, but I was acutely conscious of my cowardice about talking to my mother. Knowing that in another two years I should be twenty-five, I felt it might be better to wait until I was certain how to take my next step. I discovered that there were three beings bottled up in me. A first who was quite happy if left alone and not interfered with, a second who deliberately procrastinated and tried to ignore important things by over-exercising at games, and a third, an ambitious eager creature, yearning to be a credit to great-grandfather William Wilberforce. I decided to start by telling Dolly, under a vow of secrecy, and try to get her on my side.

I went to stay with Barbara [another sister] near Brough in East Yorkshire before returning home. She was ill in bed with bronchitis and I gave her inhalations and nursed her and insisted on dosing a young nephew of my brother-in-law's with hot cinnamon drinks to save him from catching the same infection. It seems I never lost a chance to try my hand at amateur doctoring! One day I went on a walk on my own across fields until I found myself in a beech wood. The utter silence filled my spirit with an inner peace. I spent a good time thinking and planning. Sir Thomas Browne says, 'Be able to be alone. Lose not the advantages of solitude, and the society of thyself.'

Now had come the time when I felt compelled to decide my future; *was* I born to be a bond slave to family life forever? I could do it quite well I felt sure, but was that all I needed from

33

the gift of Life? I was plainly made in a different mould from the rest of my family. That I knew. I had always felt from my own observation that women had far more practical sense and imagination than most men. Hence if not trammelled by family commitments I thought I could be a reasonably good doctor. On the other hand I had an untrained mind and found it hard to concentrate. It was fatally easy for me to be diverted by the goings-on of others. I was, in fact, too good an audience. How could I pass those stiff examinations? I left the beech wood with an iron determination not to be lazy or cowardly but to carve out my own career and study Medicine, however hard it might be.

When I reached home Janet was definitely worse. Mr Brunning, the kind postmaster in his shirt sleeves (it was a scorching hot summer in 1911), leant elegantly and confidentially over the counter and asked if I had seen Janet lately? 'She is looking very poorly. Indeed, though you wouldn't mention it to her, I feel she is in a decline.' Janet was a rare person and I really had more in common with her than with either Phyllis or Joan. Among other things she understood 'the value of solitude'.

That day at luncheon my mother discussed the Campion girls in pitying terms, saying that when their parents died they'd have little to live upon and that she didn't suppose they realised what their position would be if they didn't marry. She enumerated various young men and asked if I liked any one of them. She said that Susan and I would be left a discontented couple of old maids on a hundred or two a year. I laughed and told her to cheer up for I might die young which would save a lot of bother, but I was firmly told I was now no longer young. She then said Susan was lazy and didn't help even over garden party invitations. I teased her and said that without me she wouldn't give garden parties and have nice roses, and she would have no water, for this was one of the household jobs I was responsible for. I tried to point out the difference my absence would make until at length my mother was stung to reply, 'Don't you think you are so indispensable.'

The tragic situation caused by the delay in diagnosis over Janet galvanised me into taking my next step; and I wrote for particulars from medical schools. I was horrified to learn that Matriculation was necessary in five subjects which included Latin and Mathematics, for I knew practically nothing of either. My sister, Dolly, had advised me to talk to my mother and be open about taking the examination without specifying the reason, and this seemed a good scheme. In a letter to Miss Robins I told her of my despair at failing to get Janet's consent to go away for treatment, and that I meant to persist in my determination to become a doctor.

Miss Robins answered me at Dolly's house, Lovelands, where I was staying a few days, and where my letters were not likely to be opened. She informed me that at one moment she had

> an impression that my interest and real sense of sharing in your good or ill had received a check. . . . I was vaguely feeling: nice girl, uncommon girl but choked like a flower struggling for life in a weedy garden. And, oh black injustice! Content to be choked I thought, not really struggling up to sunshine and free air as I had believed. What use then to go caring deeply for a life like that! Waste, sheer waste of an interest that was wanted elsewhere. Well, I am perhaps glad not only for you – that you (with that old Liberator behind you) are not content with the slow choking process. I'm glad not only for you, but glad for me, that I no longer need ever wonder: is she worthwhile – this Sussex child?
>   Your friend
>   Elizabeth Robins

This was heady stuff from my hero-worshipped friend. Though I had been trained in submission it was suddenly brought home to me that I had a stake in life and above all a mind and soul of my own. I talked again to Phyllis who was full of enthusiasm and advised me to tell Miss Robins everything, but even to Phyllis I was careful not to say too much of my family trials. How carefully I was treading!

On 19 August out of a full heart I wrote a long letter to E.R., as I started to call her. I tried to express what I found it difficult to say to her face. In the written word, which I always valued more than speech, I burned my boats. However greatly I tortured myself in the next months at the thought of failure and wounding my mother, there was never again to be any going back.

I've got a lot of particulars (re examination, etc.) – they are wonderfully interesting. Being blissfully ignorant I fail to understand the immensity of the job. Suddenly to find oneself actually and incredibly in the midst of a dream come true is rather like having all the breath taken out of one by very cold water. I couldn't think – let alone talk – coherently at all.

You might remember this, so long as my family are away you will do me most good by casting many doubts on my ability to pass these examinations. Then you will make me sullenly and doggedly determined just to show you. . . . And then later if I get depressed and things seem impossible to realise, then I may say your optimism will come fresh at the right moment. So don't waste it now!

To say that I owe everything to you is perfectly true. When John was ill I first thought about doctoring; in January I talked to Phyllis about it. In March I mentioned it to you, quite unintentionally; allow me to point out that it was quite a minor act of bravery! I knew that day it would have to be done sooner or later. But the idea of Medicine was *mine*.

But though you weren't responsible for the idea, you are wholly responsible for me. It is easy to say, 'It would have happened in any case', but who knows? I'm inclined to think otherwise, but even if it had, it would have been years later and where *now* failure is a possibility, then it would have been a certainty.

For one thing you made me think that I was an individual. It wasn't that I was unselfish, I was simply *self less* before. I didn't realise, I didn't feel, I didn't trouble about anything. When John was ill one of the nurses told me I was a fool and I was to strike out for myself. That hadn't much effect. Then from talking to you came a desire to learn – Wragge found by you. And with that came more acquaintance with you and the beginning of Life. I talked to you and you always listened. That was new; as a rule people never listened, they always interrupted and I don't believe I ever said anything I really meant till I began to know you. Somehow I found I wanted to be truthful to you, and I always have wanted to be.

And then I gradually realised with much surprise that I had become very fond of you. When I was a child and all my life I had firmly determined that I would never really care about anyone or anything! I would be friendly and polite and hoped to make everybody think that I adored them but right deep down I would always know that I didn't really care a bit. So I looked upon it as an insult when I made the fatal discovery, and I fell inches, yards, in my own estimation; worse and worse, I couldn't stop caring, which surprised me yet more. However since then I've become hardened to it and the fact has to live with me – same as eating and sleeping – as a part of my existence.

But what you've done is that you've made me know that there *is* a world and in it are Joy and Sorrow, Happiness, Misery – and Friendship and a verb To Care. It is all from *you*. And now I want to help people. There is no real way of helping people, when they are worried or anxious, or of doing them any lasting help because they must help themselves, but I do want to *try* and heal and help them bodily, physically. And of course I may be no good. It is appalling to feel one can't help people. You help them tremendously with your books and they are differently disposed to things afterwards.

But now when I tell you it is all due to you, you shirk the responsibility. You too are a coward! It's all very well to say I'll care furiously for someone someday, that is only shirking responsibility too. You've said I am unlike the others of my family and it is true, and they are no help to me. I puzzle them and they puzzle me. I am *alone* and you mustn't shirk; you must accept the fact that you are the one being who I have come to care for with all the concentrated bottled up affection of twenty-three years, which with most people has been scattered about in many directions. That may be a better plan, but how can I help it?

So don't shirk and drive me back to the tepid existence I'm struggling out of. I want you *always*, whether I make an awful muddle of things, or – whatever happens, to keep a finger on me at all times and in all places.

Charlie's death was another reason, as I afterwards told Phyllis, for my obstinate resolve to get through my examinations as fast as I could and become a doctor. I felt he would have been enthusiastic about the doctoring idea for I remember he had once talked to my mother for nearly two hours on the subject of girls doing things and being *free*. She hadn't responded!

With a beating heart, I told my mother that I wanted to take Matriculation. I did not tell her the real reason, but said that I wanted to feel more educated. She was then feeling sorry for me after Charlie's death, and agreed, especially as Phyllis said that she would like to take it too, which gave a semblance of naturalness to the undertaking. Perhaps my mother thought it was a new phase among a certain type of young women. Absurd, of course, but it would keep us occupied. With Phyllis I had a long, sad talk about Charlie, which relieved our pent up feelings and drew us even closer together.

That autumn was not an easy one. It was the time of my greatest struggle over Janet and a battle with her about going into a sanatorium for treatment. It was only after much persistence on my part that she finally agreed. I found it difficult to persuade her without frightening her, for I couldn't say, 'Your case is desperate unless you have treatment.' Yet I fully realised myself from the Brompton report that in any case it was only a question of time and that she was classed as a hopeless case. All the same I knew we ought to try and see what complete rest and good food might do. It was next to impossible to find a vacancy anywhere, but at last I was lucky to get her away to a more or less private sanatorium run by a medical woman. The charges at that time were £6.7.8d a month, and E.R. helped me with the fees. Janet began to improve, her temperature settled, her cough subsided and as she gained weight and strength she naturally hankered to go home. I tried to persuade her to stay a little longer for I was also deeply concerned about the risk of infection for the baby, but she would not stay as long as I wanted her to do.

My mother was in an injured mood. She expected me to talk to her all the time about my feelings and my aims. She asked me how much E.R. knew about either and I lied and said she knew nothing, partly because I was afraid of my mother's anger and partly because Phyllis had warned me not to let her know of E.R.'s participation. Characteristically, I confessed my cowardice and lack of truth to E.R. I concentrated hard on learning about Matriculation and was also spending time over Janet. I wanted to be left alone and resented being followed about and talked to. Why was I expected to tell all that I thought and felt and did?

I had started special coaching in Latin and Mathematics with two of the staff from Roedean, again recommended by Miss Lawrence. Miss Lowenstein taught Latin to the most junior pupils and she was ideal for the virgin soil of my knowledge. Miss Rowbotham was a brilliant mathematician who made everything seem crystal clear and easy when I was with her, but on reaching home to my utter disgust I realised I understood not one word. She had to deal with rock as a seed bed for I have never grasped the elements of the exacting subject of Mathematics. They both worked hard to help me and I might have progressed more rapidly if there hadn't been incessant family interruptions to destroy my budding powers of concentration. I was constantly being lectured about my many crimes. One was 'Solemnity with increasing age', which was put down to sums! Phyllis had promised to do Matriculation with me but she bitterly disappointed me by backing out, which annoyed me.

In October [1911] I was allowed to stay at Cromer with the Buxtons. Wherever I visited I took my books with me. I was trying hard to study and it was a fruitful time for me to take stock. My awakening to the possibilities and beauties of Friendship roused me to other ideas and the desire for real work. My memories of Charlie's high ideals and longing for good conspired to urge me on.

[A few months afterwards] I was invited to go to [Gstaad in] Switzerland with Joan. I enjoyed the cheerful gay excitement, which seemed to affect Joan and me particularly, from the first impact of cherry jam and hot chocolate. Joan was an ideal companion and we were both equal beginners [at skiing] but felt we had more or less got the hang of it after a few days. It had been arranged that I should, at the end of a fortnight, join the Buxtons at St Moritz where they too were to have a winter sports holiday. I was allowed to go to St Moritz [by train] by myself. It was good to be there and I was happy. The Buxton party were not at all advanced over skiing and we had to stay around on the nursery slopes where there were huge pot-holes to avoid. I stupidly caught the toe of my ski in one and it fell under me. Something happened to my knee and I couldn't get up. It was very painful. I was taken into the hotel and a Swiss doctor was summoned who bound it up but did not reduce the dislocated semilunar cartilage – synovitis followed and I was made to rest. When I returned to Bramlands I was ordered massage, but the pain and swelling did not lessen after three weeks and I went to an orthopaedic surgeon. He was horrified by the bad treatment I had had, put me into a nursing-home and under an anaesthetic broke down adhesions, reduced the dislocated cartilage, and put me into a plaster from hip to heel.

I soon learned to heave myself into the dogcart and hoped to continue my coaching. One Sunday I was determined to go to Backset but Miss Lucy Phillimore was staying at Bramlands and she would have thought the judgment day at hand if the pony went out, so I walked the two miles, plaster and all. By now I had begun to learn how to study and was getting on. Miss Lowenstein had written to sympathise about my knee and about my father being ill. She had realised I had no hope of getting to Brighton so she offered to come over in the luncheon hour; if she could catch the 2.08 train back, Miss Lawrence would allow her to change the Roman History lesson once more. I hope I was sufficiently grateful at thus upsetting the Roedean time table! Miss Rowbotham came to my rescue in

Mathematics, having been stirred to take an interest in my project through the good offices of Miss Lowenstein. She arrived on a motor cycle, which was very advanced in 1912.

On 11 April 1912 I stayed with Uncle Basil at 20 Dean's Yard, Westminster. My mother was with me and we went to see the orthopaedic surgeon, Mr Tubby. I described my life and its annoyances in a letter to E.R.:

> I feel fat and flabby mentally, and willing to sleep all day. I hate all this luxury; it makes me feel both mentally and physically nauseated! I'm simply pining for Sussex and weeds. Tuesday I've made up my mind to return. Can't work here. Shan't try to work till I can get into a bath. My room leads into my mother's and I'm never alone. She's as happy as a king and loves London. I only long for weeds.
>
> After luncheon yesterday, as a treat, I was taken to the House of Commons to see my uncle robe himself and process with the Speaker to read prayers. He's a queer old thing. That job makes him ten years younger in the doing of it. The moment he enters the House ten years drop off him and he is erect, alert and *un*-deaf! He would live to a hundred and thirty if they turned on prayers three times a day.
>
> [Mr Tubby] was surprised at the muscular condition [of my knee] and asked what I had been doing.
>
> 'Everything, including getting in and out of a dogcart.'
>
> 'Massage for a fortnight,' he said. Nature and I were to work it gradually back. The knee felt flabby and horribly weak; I can barely walk at all but I'm going to have a bath in about an hour! I'm to take no risks this summer i.e. no games.

E.R. was greatly preoccupied with [the Women's Suffrage agitation]. 'Mrs Pankhurst in the Dock' said the placards and 'Vain Search for Christabel'. This was enough for the Henfield villagers to be convinced she was being concealed at Backset and E.R.'s correspondence was watched by the police! The Pankhursts would come to stay and were constantly seeking her advice. I usually avoided this subject [with my family] for it was a matter which always aroused antagonism. [On one occasion] E.R. came to tea at Bramlands and her diary says: 'Mr Wilberforce roars foolishly: "You'll never get the vote – Destruction of England, etc".'

I took pains to report to my family E.R.'s influential political and literary friends. Sir Frederick Pollock, the Ian Hamiltons, Lady Brassey were among those who visited her. And H.G. Wells. The family were critical of this visit. They did not know that he had invited himself, that he had stayed up till past midnight arguing with E.R., who disapproved of his affair with the daughter of one of her friends. I am sure my selection of the well-known names of that time did a little impress my family and E.R. took great pains to be on friendly terms with my mother. She sincerely admired my mother's musical compositions and encouraged her. On 16 April 1912 came news of the *Titanic* disaster and E.R. was deeply shocked to hear of the death of her devoted friend, W.T. Stead [former editor of the *Pall Mall Gazette*], who had helped to make her journey to the Klondyke possible. A disaster of this magnitude was haunting – she could think of nothing else.

My mother went to tea with E.R. 'Queer long talk' is noted in E.R.'s diary and bits of this talk came out by degrees. I learned that, 'In the South the girls all get married young and get their families over by the time they are thirty, then they can take up other interests, so Miss Robins says. Such an excellent plan.' My mother seemed to find girls difficult creatures – particularly me. I was a puzzling, worrying problem to deal with. 'The French system is so much the best and turns out so happily. The mothers meet and arrange it all.' It was plain that my mother liked E.R. and had got on with her. I felt that my mother was right in saying I was not grown up.

I wrote in June 1912, 'This is probably the happiest year of my life', because I felt I was getting on and making real headway and working five to six hours a day. In Latin I was sure I'd found my feet. In Mathematics I was also working hard and sometimes seemed to have grasped quite a bit of knowledge. But I had phases of exasperation and even desperation. I was staying with Dolly and from the moment of my arrival I felt she was all against my plans, though pretending sympathetically to encourage me. I talked sincerely on how much I enjoyed the work. She asked when I was taking my examination and whether I was still thinking of doctoring, to which I replied, 'Why, of course', and laughed with derision at any idea of having given it up.

She went on: 'What will you do when you've passed it?'

'Oh, then the family will have to be talked to. But I'm afraid I'm rather superstitious and hate discussing things until I've seen whether I have any intelligence and until I have passed.'

[Dolly did not think the family would permit it.] 'If you were my daughter I shouldn't let you. It's such hard work and for so long; you see, for seven years you couldn't do anything else.'

[I responded that] one need never be afraid of hard work. Considering our ancestors had such terrific energy and power for good, wasn't it about time that one of the family made an attempt to follow in their footsteps? She might be shocked, surprised, annoyed, but I thought it would be fun. I shifted the discussion on to how to sell some shares of which, on John's advice, I had bought £100 worth. They had fallen disastrously but I wanted the cash to pay for my tuition. She offered to lend me £2 or £3 which I did not accept. She said I must come to her on 16 June to help entertain Mr Webster. It was plain they had planned that Mr Webster, through marrying me, should put a stop to my wild ambitions.

About this time I wrote one long depressed letter to E.R.:

There is only one thing I know and that is that the sooner I get away from here the better. I'm going to write you a letter that you'll please burn and forget because it is going to complain in a way that makes me ashamed. We'll begin with Tuesday: I arranged with endless manoeuvring two successive lessons. Miss Rowbotham was tired, saw it in her eye; also saw that I, being stupid, was trying her patience. Result – I was more stupid. Struggled with endless ordering of books, etc. from the University Correspondence College, giving me instructions in English, French and History. Wednesday:

Everything one does is wrong – oh, incredibly wrong. I interview Mrs Rodgers and order suitable food which at any ordinary time would be specially appreciated – all wholly wrong.

Thursday afternoon: I got half-an-hour, seized the Algebra and found I had not remembered one single thing Miss Rowbotham had told me. Then I lost my temper with myself and Fate in general. The waste of time and money and trouble of having a lesson and one's gaining nothing – it was too much. Then I have to write down the washing – which is Susan's job by rights – have no time for even a glass of milk and dash off to Lowenstein. Tired? No. Cross? Yes, very.

In June 1912 E.R. gave a party at the Writers Club for some of her literary friends, both English and American, and she was kind enough to invite me. It was a boiling hot day and all sorts of writers were there. I had to have a frock and a hat and white gloves, and I handed cakes and absorbed the appearance of the guests. They were not the least as I had imagined. Then E.R. took me by the arm and introduced me to Mrs Yates Thompson, a big smiling, kind-faced, handsome woman with most attractive greenish eyes under a large hat. Where did I live and what did I do, she asked. 'Aren't all these literary worthies alarming? I've really no claim to be here at all,' she went on. Was I fond of music, and would I ever care to go to an opera with her? I was thrilled at the prospect of an opera. I had only been to one or two. When the party was over I told E.R. about the possible opera and asked who Mrs Yates Thompson was.

'She's one of my dearest friends, the eldest daughter of George Smith, the publisher of the Brontes and Thackeray.'

I interrupted and told her that Mrs Yates Thompson had said she had no claim to be there, at which E.R. chuckled. 'How like her shy modesty – more right to be there than many of them.' When I returned home with a full report of my new acquaintance my family were rather impressed.

A week later came the invitation for the opera. I had nothing suitable for such an occasion so I had to get a new evening dress and my mother insisted on long white gloves. I stayed with Aunt Betty. I was much excited and dreadfully shy, the more so as I was conducted up the wide imposing staircase at 19 Portman Square by the grave, perfectly-mannered butler, Parsons, and was announced into a large drawing-room with beautiful pictures and glass cases containing treasures. [There were four or five other guests, including Mr Le Fanu, the H.A.L. Fishers, and 'Haggy']—Mr Hagberg Wright of the London Library. Mr Le Fanu had kindly, reassuring manners and understood what was expected of him in dealing with an out-of-her-depth young country woman. After the sumptuous dinner and the perfection of first-class service I was carefully handed in to the brougham with its spanking horses and a footman on the box, with two other women and our hostess, the rest of the party following in taxis. The whole evening was breathtaking, the opera divine.

I was asked again, but most delightful of all, I was asked for a weekend at Oving, their country house near Aylesbury. Mrs Thompson met me at Waddesdon Manor Station in a high dogcart and she was wearing a country tweed coat and skirt and a wide-brimmed, well-worn Panama hat. She told me how before marriage she had longed to join her father in publishing. If she had been a son this would have been easy; as a daughter she could only help unofficially. I encouraged her to talk of her early days, how she loved riding with Trollope and what a dear kind man he was. The Brontes, Thackeray, Dicky Doyle and Leech of *Punch*, George du Maurier, all came into her memories. In my young enthusiasm, and if it were not for Medicine, I wished I could go into publishing with her.

There was a high walled garden with rampant fig trees, violets in frames, peaches in glasshouses and huge asparagus beds. There was a billiard room and everywhere wonderful books. The lighting was from candles and lamps, and one felt the whole household ran on oiled wheels. I was taken and shown the pedigree Jersey cows of which I knew absolutely nothing. But Mrs Thompson had a great eye for their points and the Jersey bull was brought out by Jesson, the herdsman, and paraded in front of us. I had never enjoyed a weekend so much and was invited again later on. After dinner we often played billiards. I

45

had not played since Lavington days but I loved the game. One Sunday night I was very lucky and beat Mr Hagberg Wright. He was brother to Sir Almroth Wright and as strongly anti-feminist. Mr Thompson couldn't resist the temptation to tease him mercilessly. He chuckled and chuckled: 'Fancy Haggy being beaten by the grand-daughter of her saponaceous relative [Bishop Samuel Wilberforce – "Soapy Sam"] – beaten by a *girl*.' And his eyes twinkled wickedly with glee as he rubbed it in. Haggy was so annoyed that he could hardly bring himself to say goodnight to me. I felt I had achieved fame!

Other people seem to wish for society to let off their bad temper on. My one desire is solitude and permission to wallow in a book. Then I recover and come out fresh as one does after bathing in the sea.

4

THE FAMILY
AGAINST MEDICINE

1912–13

In spite of coaching by Miss Lowenstein and Miss Rowbotham
I made slow progress. The leg in plaster was a source of frus-
tration which I thought I had borne with some equanimity, but
Joan told me that I had been quite unbearable. During the
spring and summer of 1912 I paid many visits, to Aunt Betty
and Dolly in London, to Danny, to the Bouveries, to Barbara
in Yorkshire, and then the Buxtons in Scotland. And though I
found it easier to work at the Buxtons – in fact almost anywhere
better than at Bramlands – it was not good for study to be so
much on the move. When I was thoroughly depressed on one
occasion I had gone to Backset and found it far easier to concentrate and work there – partly because E.R.'s friendly presence
put fresh heart into me and I felt she was behind me in all my
efforts. Boldly overcoming my diffidence I told her this: 'Then
you can never have any excuse because I'm always there,' she
replied in a reassuring voice. I was stirred to fresh efforts by
the memory of those words and I determined I must not fail
her.

E.R.'s friend, Dr Louisa Martindale, to whom I was
immensely grateful for having diagnosed Janet, was busy trying
to raise funds to start a hospital in Brighton for women patients,
to be staffed only by medical women. I boldly undertook to
organise a concert in Henfield for this worthwhile object. Little
did I realise all it involved. We got Helen Mar, Effie Cooke of
the Follies, who was a great draw, Lady Sybil Smith and others.
There were two performances to packed and appreciative audiences and we proudly handed over £40 as a contribution

47

towards the beginning of what subsequently became the New Sussex Hospital.

I loved my visit to the Bouveries at High Barn near Godalming, as not only was Dorothy a lovable person and very kind to me, but she played the piano beautifully. Dorothy played Brahms with a tenderness and understanding that enthralled me. She confided in me her medical adventures with no less than eleven doctors, all of whom she had finally shaken off after they had failed to help her. She had developed a philosophy of her own and kept her sense of humour.

When I came back from High Barn in November 1912 I told my mother the reason why I wanted to take Matriculation. She said nothing much at the time and it is possible that Dolly had hinted at my wish to study Medicine; but as soon as John arrived on the scene my mother felt fortified to express her adamant refusal to allow me to do this. Among other things it was 'unsexing'. They had no objection, she said, to my becoming a nurse. On this score I had an answer, for a nurse was far more intimately concerned with a patient and in fact was with him all the time, whereas a doctor only visited. They were not unduly troubled as they thought I had not the brains to pass the examinations, nor the physical stamina for the hard work involved in the seven years study. These arguments had curiously little effect on my resolve; in fact they only made me twice as determined to carry on and show them what I could do. I was like a plant hardening off.

On 12 December E.R. decided that she must go to New York to negotiate about her new book. Characteristically rapid, she sailed two days later. Her departure coincided with information from my coaches that I had no chance if I tried for Matriculation in January. Obstinately I thought the experience might be helpful; moreover a hundred to one chance can be more exciting than a two to one, and I have always enjoyed gambling. E.R.'s leaving was a wrench and I accompanied her in the train as far as Horsham. When I returned to Bramlands I was questioned as to why I was so late, to which I replied that I wanted to talk to her – said with a fire of truth and firmness that astonished both parties about equally.

Apart from my difficulties over work and Miss Rowbotham's discouragement I was worried about money. I was overdrawn £10.11.9d. My tuition fees came to £15 and the University Correspondence College would be about £4. I was determined I would not borrow from Dolly and I was doubtful if I could face tackling my mother. Could I risk the bank not returning my cheques? Had I better write to my kind coaches and ask if they would mind waiting – perhaps they had already bought Christmas presents out of my lessons? It was all very complicated. My mother, by way of encouragement, told me I had never looked so tired. I knew I had no hope of passing – not even in one subject, but I still hoped the experience would be useful. Miss Lowenstein explained to me that this was the only examination which can't be crammed. The University Correspondence College sent me a report on 18 December: 'English and French: on border line between success and failure. Effective revision imperative.' And these were my best subjects!

When I went to stay with Aunt Betty for the examination I was desperately tired. I had resigned myself that I could not pass even in English and was in consequence depressed. By the last day, when there was French in the morning and Modern History in the afternoon, I was nearly at the end of my resources. I went to lunch with the Rendels, for which I had altogether from 1 to 2.30 p.m., and was just starting my meal when Susan rang me up and asked me to go down and keep my father company for the afternoon. I wrote an indignant account of this family thoughtlessness to E.R. and went on to describe my visit:

One word about my visit here – I'm very susceptible to kindness and they have all been kind to me – Betty most of all, of course, but Jack and Mark have both been awfully kind. 'How have you got on today?' they both say the moment we meet after a fresh paper, and so I give them the paper to look at and explain how badly I've done and they're so interested. They may think I'm mad to do it, and they look at me with a wondering gaze, but they've never said they see no good in it and they both encourage me. I'm so grateful and unused to it, it is very strange to me!

The invigilator came to me this morning and asked me how I was getting on, having puzzled all night, I expect, as to why I was allowed to enter with the ideas of Latin that she saw yesterday. I said, 'Oh, *hopelessly*, thanks very much. You see I've never been in for any examinations before, and I've only been working in it for a year.'

'Only a year; well of course, it's quite absurd,' said she. She's quite a nice creature and hovered round all day and sat near me, furtively watching my bewildered expression and futile endeavour!

When I returned to Bramlands I felt the existing conditions to be bad for my work as well as vile for my character. I persisted in trying to take Matriculation from there in spite of continual harassing, in the hope that my family would finally come round and accept as inevitable the future I had chosen. I excused myself to E.R., who had not approved, by saying:

Never again will I try to take a middle course, it's worse than walking on a tight rope. The anti-doctoring, anti-women stream was continuously poured on my unoffending head [by my mother and John]. I have been hearing a great deal about women lately. No sense of honour, no sense of humour and a very great deal more to the effect that they are a miserable infliction on the world, and that every normal girl in a room containing fifteen women and one man would wish to attract and talk to the one man. I must be terribly abnormal as my natural instinct is to avoid having to talk to male or female!

A Miss Collie who is the head of Bedford High School predicts that I shall never pass the Matriculation. One must be properly educated to do so, from the beginning. So that's encouraging for you! When I reported this to Miss Rowbotham she said I *was* attempting a very great deal and would have to work at Mathematics alone for three hours a day if I hope to make any show at all in June.

Shortly after this Phyllis and I arrived at the London School of Medicine in Hunter Street. I asked to see Miss Louie M. Brooke and sent in my name. After five minutes of great trepidation we were shown into a nice airy room where a woman was sitting at the table writing. She rose and shook us warmly by the hand and said, 'Oh you've come to see our school. Do you both want to be doctors?' We explained hurriedly that I was the culprit. She told us that after about three years one begins hospital work as well as the theoretical work. There was only accommodation for sixteen students at the school, for which there was a great demand, but many were taken in by women doctors and boarded while they were being trained. The cost for the seven years, and board and lodging at school or at various hostels close by, came to £1000. There were nine hundred women qualified in England as against thirty thousand men. Many of the former were abroad. The ones at home were engaged chiefly in public work and did not have private practices. They were much needed in the country, lamentably so, she said, but they couldn't make a living. They constantly get requests from small country towns for women doctors but they would starve if they went, so they have to stick to large towns. A country doctor would have to have private means. Most students start at twenty or twenty-one years old. Then she showed us over the school, and when she said goodbye added that she hoped to see me again in October.

One evening after I got home my mother came into my room to talk to me. 'I am very unhappy about you and your examination,' she said. 'If you are still thinking of being a doctor, you'd better give it up at once. The whole thing is unpractical. For one thing you're too old. The profession is already overcrowded and hundreds of girls are going into it from the North, further overcrowding it. Besides, you would have to live in London. You are too young to live in London.'

'Just now you said I was too old, and now I'm too young,' I remarked. And I added that Dr Martindale had told me the supply didn't meet the demand and all the women doctors she knew were doing well.

'Women are so inaccurate, I don't believe her,' said my

mother. 'But as regards the living in London and the training, I tell you at once and finally I couldn't afford it, so that's the end of it. I spend everything I have on making your father's remaining years happy and deprive myself of many pleasures in doing so. If you are thinking of doing it to make a living you will only starve. And you are to understand that if anything happened to us, you and Susan would have a little money to live on, enough to make it unnecessary for you to have to make a living.'

I was hating the whole conversation, but keeping very calm and firm and cool. [My mother continued:] 'Also it wants great physical strength and you aren't at all strong; look at the throats you get.'

'Really, I don't think anyone could term me unsound,' and I laughed with scorn.

'Also it means five or six years.'

'Yes,' I interrupted, 'and isn't that a short time when one thinks of what one is fitted for, at the end?' A horribly disconcerting remark for my opponent!

'Well, and then you would be wasting the best years of your youth and happiness – you would lose all your friends. Why see, already the Campions haven't asked you to stay lately, simply on account of your being so engrossed and stupid about your work.'

I said I thought they had but I had generally refused.

'You would be sure to break down; even now you get sometimes to look so careworn that you make me dreadfully unhappy about you. You would be mixing solely with girls of a lower class. The majority would be much beneath you. You couldn't possibly do anything socially, and you would ruin your chance of a woman's only real happiness – being a mother. I should be very sorry about that and I feel sure you would regret it later. You would only be allowed to attend women, and in the country it would only be very ordinary ailments like colds. It would be a very dull life. Doll's is a most interesting life. And she has the satisfaction of knowing that she is making one man perfectly happy.' Then she went off into a lecture on the happiness to be obtained from a marriage for money.

'If you feel you want to do good, you can do more good by living at home and making your parents happy than in any other way. What does Miss Robins say?' I hedged on this as Phyllis had advised; she thought E.R.'s approval would antagonise my mother still more. John had been written to and I supposed he would next be turned on to bully me.

In due course the results of Matriculation came through. I had of course failed. But there was one surprise. I had actually passed in English. My knowledge of grammar was nil; I was bad at trying to write a précis. The University Correspondence College had never liked the way I tried to write an essay, but it was the essay which earned the highest marks. I remember I enjoyed writing it and the examiner must have felt lenient when he read it. English was the only subject in the Matriculation examination at which I never failed. The family continued their old tactics.

It was really most foolish to try for Matriculation in June but it did help me even though I was warned I had no chance. The Buxtons were very kind and allowed me to stay at 5 Buckingham Gate for six weeks intensive work with Mr Pierpoint, a much-vaunted mathematical coach. This gave me an opportunity to experience what a difference it made to work uninterruptedly in an encouraging atmosphere. They themselves were not there very much, only coming up for a night or so at intervals. On one occasion I was greatly touched by Mr Buxton's kindness. He was up for the night and not only insisted on breakfasting at an earlier hour than was his wont, in order to share it with me, but he himself rearranged the table and the light in the way he thought would be most comfortable for my work. As the busiest Minister in the Liberal Government (at that time he was in charge of the Board of Trade) he must have been more appreciative of my aims than I had imagined.

People were certainly very kind to me in my few breaks from work. Mrs Yates Thompson asked me to dine and go to a concert. Later on she wrote: 'A very clever little American friend of ours, Ruth Draper, is going to do some monologues for us. I wish you would come and hear her.' I was dreadfully shy, as I knew hardly a soul in the crowded gathering and everybody was marvellously gowned. I was spellbound by Ruth Draper. When it was all over a portentous figure rose to his feet, everybody made way for him, and I sensed that this was some Great Man indeed. He flung out his arms and made admiring Great Phrases with immense enthusiasm. I saw Mrs Yates Thompson's face beam with delight. Ruth had indeed brought it off – and Ruth herself was overjoyed and her dark eyes flashed at his warm praise. I asked a neighbour who this was and was told with almost withering scorn, 'Oh, but Mr Henry James.' Mrs Yates Thompson later in the evening introduced me to Ruth Draper and I stammered something of the admiration which overwhelmed me then, as ever after.

After I had failed the examination again – always in Mathematics – I stayed with Aunt Betty and she took me over the East End Lying-in-Home for Mothers in Stepney. Mrs Anderson, the Matron, was a friend of Aunt Betty's and had been told about me, and her enthusiasm cheered me on. The mothers were cheerful, smiling and joking. They told me how much they looked forward to the one fortnight's rest they enjoyed in the year. A woman of forty-five had died the previous day with her *nineteenth* child. She was worn out physically. Since her leaving the Home last year she had only been out of the house once, which was the day she had come to book a bed. In a letter to E.R. I said: 'And then one talks of enlightenment, education, progress, civilisation. My God.'

To say I was discouraged about the examination is unnecessary. I was still determined, although I began to doubt whether I had the necessary brains to get through. I wrote to Miss Rowbotham, knowing that she would tell me the truth. Her answer, written on 1 July 1913, was balm to my shattered confidence:

> There isn't anything the matter with your brains in my opinion. Your difficulties arise from the fact that your mind is not as plastic as it was before you were grown up. You see all these things you are learning now ought to have been learned when you were growing, and in that case the effort of memory would not have been so great. I don't know

whether this statement is psychologically true but I think it is. I do think that you have undertaken a big task in trying to make up for lost time but I don't think you need despair and I certainly think you have got your share of brains right enough.

After a good deal of negotiation with the authorities I was allowed to start at the London School of Medicine for Women on condition that I worked for the January Matriculation. In that way I should not lose a whole year as the first medical teaching always began in October. The curriculum was Chemistry, Biology and Physics. It was not a good plan, as I enjoyed the pre-medical classes and only brought a rather tired brain to the burdensome Matriculation work. However I think it was Mr Pierpoint who suggested I might try for the College of Preceptors examination, as he thought I should get through that all right. He may have imagined that it would get me over my examination fears.

I was worried about where to stay for the beginning of the term. Aunt Betty could not have me and I wrote to consult E.R. She was cautious in her reply and said she could not gauge the Bramlands situation and would not like to advise. But she finished her letter by saying she always felt happier about my ability to work when I was with the Buxtons. They themselves fully realised how true this was. The attitude of my family was as unrelenting as ever. I felt I had to share my feelings with Phyllis, who answered with a comforting letter:

People are being stupid and not understanding about one another. There is an immense gulf fixed, I know, between you and your family about women. Your family will never allow that what is sauce for the gander is sauce for the goose, and from their point of view they are right. That gulf is always going to remain, but I do think it might be bridged over. It's so unbearable like this. Your mother must be dreadfully unhappy too; oh I do wish I could talk to her. Do you think she won't ever see me again? Is Aunt Betty standing by you? It will be very great of her if she does and all my hope is on her.

I wish you could be comforted and they could be comforted – me too. I feel all battered. Is it much to you that I believe in you with all my heart and soul? Perhaps that's why I mind for them so much, because though they are right, you are righter.

Phyllis was most anxious to tackle any of my relations who were being obstructive. She had promised to pay for my tuition and examination fees but she startled me by saying she had not yet told her father about this.

Modern parents must think it incredible that daughters were so scared of their parents. Since my family strongly disapproved of my wanting to take a medical training there was a plain reason for refusal. But with Phyllis who 'doated' – to use her own word – on her father and had herself a comfortable allowance, was it a matter for discussion whether she should contribute £40 yearly to my fees? Our fear of family disapproval has already been indicated by the insistence on the part of Joan and me on keeping secret our endeavour to learn something of nineteenth-century writers. If we had enjoyed the fury of today's Angry Young, the girls of 1913 might have started a movement to emancipate young women from Slavery to Family! The First World War was to do much to make people realise that girls were capable of standing unsupported on their own feet and of determining for themselves the direction they should take.

5
MEDICAL SCHOOL FOR WOMEN
An Obstacle Course
1913–15

The Buxtons had arranged for me to stay at 5 Buckingham Gate for my first term at the London School of Medicine for Women in October 1913. E.R. agreed to come to the Opening Day. It was rather alarming as the great Common Room was filled with students of every size, shape and age, all milling round as crowded as sheep in a fold. We shook hands with Mrs Garrett Anderson, who was white-haired and gracious, and who said something tactful about William Wilberforce's great work for the slaves. I was followed by [a student nicknamed] the 'April Baby', who kept us much amused by her comments. Her entry to the Medical School, we gathered, had been the idea of her mother, Countess von Arnim, the authoress of *Elizabeth and Her German Garden*. When the April Baby returned home that night she looked up Wilberforce in *Who's Who*, and complained to me the next day that she could find nobody of that name who had to do with the White Slave Traffic. I explained that William Wilberforce had something to do with the abolition of the Slave *Trade* and she was greatly disappointed. She was a pretty, blue-eyed, fair, charming girl, small and graceful; she was paired off with a very large and cheerful blonde called Fawsett, who had excellent brains and helped the April Baby in her struggles. They became bosom friends and kindred, giggling spirits.

Most of the girls were younger than I was and of varied types. Some of them by doing Medicine were following in a parent's footstep; some had a definite urge, like myself, to be of use to the community. These were subdivided into those who wished to be medical missionaries and those who had worked in the Suffrage movement; the latter had learned a good deal about women's restricted activities, and how few opportunities there were for them to use their abilities in any other way than as ancillary to men. A few felt that if they were once qualified there was no chance of starving.

I did my best to collect all the necessary text books and instruments and was thrilled by the interest of it all. The teachers were determined to mould us into hard-working students and budding medical women, and some of my year really went ahead and gave them nothing but satisfaction. Not so myself. I was still trying to get through Matriculation, having passed in all the other subjects but Mathematics. But each time I failed I had to take the examination again in all five subjects, Mathematics and Latin being compulsory for Medicine.

Life at the School of Medicine was not one I looked forward to, for I hated London and detested herds of girls and new people. No one ever disliked the prospect of being thrown into community life for six whole years so much as I did, but I realised it was a great opportunity. I wrote to beg Miss Robins to come and see me soon, adding that it was 'bad for me with my hysterical temperament to be thwarted'. In pencil on my letter she wrote against this, 'A joke. No young woman I ever knew more steady of nerve and temper.' (I only find this in 1961!).

On 16 October 1913 E.R. sailed for the United States of America and I was feeling very forlorn. Fawsett asked me to sit next to her at lunch and asked why I looked worried. 'It's that old Matriculation – come and tell me all about it.'

'But what will you do if you fail?' asked the April Baby. Fawsett squashed her for being tactless. I made some gently mocking remark about Fawsett's massive size. She liked being ragged and in emergencies I had found that personal remarks set off the April Baby giggling helplessly while Fawsett tried to think up a good repartee.

By degrees I grew accustomed to the school life though it was strenuous. My lunch at the school consisted of hot lamb

4d, mint sauce, potatoes 1d, and cheesecake 1d. The cheesecake was a mistake. Bread 1d, butter 1d, cheese 1d (and the butter was excellent), would be my next choice. Before I left Bramlands I had been told not to spend more than 4d on my lunches and that I mustn't slack any more. They said if I hadn't wasted so many afternoons with Miss Robins I should have passed my examination. I was accused of putting my family under a great obligation to the Buxtons, which they found very unpleasant; my two sisters would have paid for me if I hadn't offended them. They asked if Phyllis had undertaken to pay all my expenses – it would cost £1500 or £2000 to become qualified. I was told I must work steadily, not go to theatres nor go away for weekends. I should not be given money for anything but work, for I couldn't live in two worlds.

I was constantly in despair over Mathematics and began to feel I should never master the simplest sum. But I enjoyed Chemistry, and I liked Biology, except for the smells of dogfish and rabbit. Of these I wrote to E.R.:

> I spent the entire day yesterday with my head over, and hands in, a rabbit's inside. Do you know the smell? Many people won't touch it but I'm very brave about that – but I do hate the smell, because when one gets home one tastes and smells nothing but rabbit! However I wasn't the least bit affected by it which is all to the good. Nor did I dream about it.

Miss Laycock, biologist, was exceptionally kind and encouraging and I had private coaching from her. She strongly advised me to take Botany instead of History in Matriculation and I thought this over and agreed. I liked her and discovered that she bought roses at auctions in the city, which showed she had a human side. She was tall, angular, dark, direct and conscientious, but so horribly clever and quick that I wanted to ask her to slow down for my less active brain. She seemed to be amused by my remarks when I answered horrible questions in class; and, because I would say when I didn't understand, I thought she liked me.

I summoned courage and asked her to be frank and tell me if she thought me very stupid. She laughed and said she certainly would. And then after a long pause, waiting in the rain for the arrival of the motor bus, she said, emphatically, 'If you want to be encouraged I will tell you what Miss Widdows said about you.' (Miss Widdows was in charge of the Chemistry work.) 'She said that of the students who had never done Chemistry before, she thought you the most intelligent.' I was cheered by Miss Laycock's telling me that and felt she had been born into this world on purpose to help me. Though I arrived home wet through, my inner warmth of encouragement carried me a long way. I felt set up and rich. Of course it might have been only because I looked intelligent and didn't go to sleep in lectures, as I told Miss Laycock, but this she didn't allow.

My father came up one day and lunched with Aunt Betty. He said I was a fool and would never get on, as I knew no sums and never would be able to do them. And he disapproved of all women doctors. I might have been depressed if Miss Laycock hadn't given me a sheaf of Botany notes, explained the headings and made me feel cheerful because it seemed easy. For the moment I felt less alarmed at the thought of that Matriculation than I had for a long time. So much depends on confidence in all examinations that if I felt tolerably happy about Botany I might get on better in other subjects.

In November 1913 I wrote a long letter to E.R. in Florida:

Mrs Buxton was very anxious that I should go and talk to Uncle Basil about my plans and difficulties with my family. So I went to see him and I told him a good deal.

'If you were my daughter I should be so very proud of you. Its the finest profession in the world, the one in which there is most self sacrifice and helping of others. They can't in these days, with a young woman of twenty-five, expect her to be content to be coddled up in cotton wool at home, *now* when women are outstripping men in every way.'

I remember we held each other's hands a lot of the time – and at these remarks I stroked him affectionately! Perhaps I was trying to cultivate the sympathy and gentleness of manner so necessary in dealing with the sick! Then he asked whether I was quite sure, and I made him convinced about that.

'I think you've learnt how to be firm in the last two years, your face has altered, it's longer from here to here. That means firmness. Now how can I help you, shall I write to them? But I don't advise that. People generally resent intervention especially from relations. They might say, "Very well, I'll stop your allowance and cut you off altogether." '

'They don't give me an allowance.'

'But how do you live?' – he was completely amazed. I told him Phyllis was paying for my tuition. We agreed that if he were to see my family he would say how proud *he* would be.

Uncle Basil was dressed in his long red cassock and his skin had become very wrinkled and seemed to hang in folds over a skeleton – nothing more. His next 'case' was a slim girl, younger than I, whose hand he was also holding, rather pretty too.

After that I went to see Dolly, as I had been told to by the Buxtons and Aunt Betty. No change to be had there. She told me that a stray doctor on Shoreham golf course had told my father that he couldn't live long. Father had become nervous about his heart in consequence, so he is being taken to Huxley on Tuesday. John was there, but he refused to meet my eye, talked to Dolly exclusively, quoted 'dear old Almroth Wright' and generally tried to make me feel in disgrace. Quite unabashed, I suggested Dolly should give me a microscope as a Christmas and brithday present for future years all in one. Cost £7.10.od. This was Phyllis's idea! But Dolly bluntly said she wouldn't, and suggested I should hire one – another person convinced of my breaking down? It was discouraging as I had no money to buy one myself.

E.R. returned on 19 December and I met her at Euston. She was feeling critical of the Buxtons because of Sydney's anti-Suffrage views. They had asked her for the usual Christmas Eve party. I was most worried that these two good friends of mine should not drift apart and I wrote urgently to beg her to reconsider:

> One thing is rather worrying me. You said you didn't want to go to the Buxtons; if this is from political motives, must it be so? They are devoted to you and they are good friends to us, oh heavens yes! I have never been able to sympathise fully with the point of view that carries politics into personal relationships. Sydney Buxton is [a Cabinet Minister] but no one could ever have expected that he would take a strong line about anything. Therefore he shouldn't be punished for not doing things for which he hasn't the capability. Do please think about it in this way before you write. You expect too much of people, I believe, but you only have to know him a little to abandon any expectation! Frankness and truth are the things that matter most. With you I'll never do anything but say what I think.

I suppose I did influence her, and thank heaven diplomatic relations were not broken off, because she suddenly received an urgent letter from Mrs Buxton to say they both wanted to see her at once. [Octavia learned later] that my father had written to the Buxtons, more or less disclaiming any further interest in me as a daughter, and asking what Sydney was proposing to do about me and my foolish determination to study Medicine.

[On 29 December Sydney Buxton replied to Mr Wilberforce's 'fierce letter' as follows:]

> Last spring when Mrs Wilberforce was talking over with my wife the question of your daughter being in London in the autumn in order to carry out her studies, my wife told Mrs Wilberforce that if it would make her mind easier, she would gladly have your daughter at Buckingham Gate for the necessary time. Mrs Wilberforce appeared to be obliged by the offer: and it was therefore arranged. I should not like to propose that your daughter should shorten her time at

Buckingham Gate which was to be till about the middle of January.

As regards your question, I was not proposing to assume the responsibility for all the expenses incidental to lodging and study; tho' *I* should be glad to do anything *I* could do for your daughter at any time.

On New Year's Eve I wrote to E.R.:

Says my mother: 'When do you go back to London and for how long?' I explain.

'To Buckingham Gate? I think you'll find they won't keep you there; when they come up they'll get rid of you. So then when they turn you out you will come home.'

'Oh no, live somewhere else.'

My mother says furiously, 'You can't live in London alone. Besides you've got no money.'

I say nonchalantly, 'Oh well, have to collect some, I expect. It costs something wherever I live,' which is about the nearest *I'll* ever get to asking them for money. Then I was lectured on my extravagance.

After Christmas I received a profound shock. For 4 January E.R.'s diary says: 'Murder's out. The Wilberforces have told Octavia of the exchange of letters between Reg Wilberforce and Sydney. Octavia outraged at her father's action.'

My birthday was on 8 January 1914 and I received an odd collection of letters from various members of my family. They were all on the same theme – the knowledgeable folk who had reported that no medical woman could ever make a living. My mother added, 'I still hope that one of these days you will look upon us as your best friends, *who by their opposition*, are making it possible for you to retire gracefully and to tell those who are backing you up that you are not continuing this course, out of deference to the wishes of your cruel parents!' I sent a selection of the family letters to E.R. and wondered how to answer them. Each letter stressed that it was very hard work and that I should certainly starve. I admitted the force of these

63

arguments. I realised that it wasn't light work and that to see people only when they are suffering would be gloomy, but, all the same, I thought that I could do it.

It was not an encouraging atmosphere to escape from to Buckingham Gate and I felt like a criminal to be deserting my family but I was determined to go on. I wrote and begged E.R. to lend me a book. 'Should I tackle a Henry James?' (she had just been seeing him). Or, 'I'm not sure I wouldn't like an Ibsen in which you played. So long as it's engrossing, compelling and preferably gloomy I'll be very happy.' She sent me *The Master Builder*, which I at once read and adored, and a cheque for £2.2.od which I decided to spend partly on taxis to the examination. Uncle Basil told me to keep him posted as to how I got on, adding, 'I will think of you daily. I am very seedy but all is well.'

The Matriculation examination began on 12 January and I wrote to E.R.:

I've not worked up the English, this is mostly your subject! Most people go in for examinations thoroughly equipped as regards education and knowledge necessary, and thoroughly equipped as regards self-confidence – having frequently done them before from an early age.

I have no equipment of necessary knowledge, no foundations. I have no equipment of self-confidence. Therefore I have to go in armed with: (1) common sense (2) nerves kept in hand by determination (3) stray disorderly fragments of knowledge.

The first day of English I was in despair and I sent the paper to my literary friend and worked off some of my rage about the ways of examiners. After it was all over I went down to Backset for the night knowing I must have failed, and then on to Bramlands.

My father was now desperately ill and he died two days later on 19 January 1914 at seventy-three years of age. I was plunged into a world of telephone messages, food arrangements, and the care of the family, most of whom were squeezed into the house, including the doctor who slept there the last night. But brother John said I created a calm atmosphere, which was handsome of him.

I had thought that at Christmas time I might tackle my family and say gently but firmly that, though I had to do things they didn't like, I was sure that one day they would see differently. Meanwhile lack of residence, food, and money was not going to prevent me from carrying out my purpose. I would have added that I thought they might try to do something for me rather than let me be wholly dependent on others. But the Buxton crisis, my birthday letters, and my failure at Matriculation prevented such an action. With my father's death there was no change in their attitude. Instead I had a terrible interview which I described to E.R. on 14 February 1914:

This has been worse than anything. John and my mother had me in to the smoking-room and gave me a 'dressing down'. Oh Lord. All my family held the same views and would always hold the same views of disapproving of my project and therefore would never help me.

[They] thought the Buxtons had behaved disgracefully. What did they mean by all this encouragement and going against my parents' wishes – which had been very expressly explained to them – and then not being thoroughly responsible, not saying 'Oh well, I'll see you through with it', but merely offering me an impossible £300 where at least £1200 (for the six years) was wanted. Most ungentlemanly, mean behaviour and they'd like to tell the Buxtons what they think. No girl, no *lady* could live on £100 a year in London, nor £140 either. Must be at least £200 and then very uncomfortably after the luxury to which I'd been accustomed. God knows how I felt. I do hope to God they don't write the Buxtons more letters.

Why did I want to be a doctor? Money? Proved idiotic. To be of use? Greatest use in staying at home and making my mother's few remaining years happy. Wouldn't have me living alone in London, put their foot down. Girls who said they lived on less than £200 lied, or else they obtained money

65

in unladylike ways. John knew. Up and down and round they rattled out arguments. I was silent to almost everything. I was so flabbergasted and taken by surprise. Much they said *was* fairly sound from their point of view.

Now it's an awful time this to have to go through and I don't quite see how we're going to get out of it without their offending the Buxtons. Damned awkward for me, altogether. And I'm most terribly sorry. Now, it's all very beastly and I've no idea how to thank you for the things you said today, but to be very brief my opinion is this. If they have to be told that I'll be paid for after the three years by you – and it's the devil that you should have to help me – I think it would be infinitely best if you tell them that yourself, not write it. Then perhaps at last they may take it as hopeless to try to stop me or starve me out.

Now, this is a loathsome letter containing bad news. I said I was an 'endless trouble' in the letter you saw to my mother. I am indeed that a hundred times over to *you*, and you probably think I'm not grateful, that I take things for granted. Listen to me, no one all the world over has ever felt as I feel, grovellingly grateful, miserably uncomfortable and dreadfully burdened with responsibility. But I look on far ahead to when I hope to be able to look back on some success and say to you, 'All this is yours, without you there would never have been anything.' If I fail you'll think of how much valuable time, money, affection you have wasted on a worthless object – naturally I'm overcome with my responsibilities.

When I returned to Buckingham Gate and my studies, further shocks awaited me. Phyllis wrote me a private letter to say that her father had been appointed Governor-General of South Africa, and they would all be going out in the spring or early summer. This was a great blow. They had been such unflinching stalwart allies, always ready to advise and support me in my struggles. Then came news of my Matriculation failure. Mathematics, every time, let me down.

Once again I was in a thoroughly depressed state. My father had cut me out of his will, my mother would only undertake, as before, to dress me, and with Sydney Buxton's departure I would lose that supporting family. But in spite of this it cannot be too firmly asserted that I had the staunchest of friends. I had received a letter from Phyllis saying that the Buxtons would allow me £100 a year for three years and Phyllis undertook to pay my fees, £40 yearly. That gave me three years of security in which to prove myself. My family were furious at the Buxton contribution, 'which should have been £1200 or nothing,' they said, and they wanted to withdraw permission for me to continue my studies. Indeed they did withdraw it and I felt shattered, but was asked for the night to Backset where I was comforted and encouraged. It was then that E.R. told me she had promised Sydney Buxton that after three years she would, if necessary, see me through. This indeed gave me fresh courage; the race against time lost some of its nightmare quality.

I carried on at the School of Medicine and wasted no time on trying to make friends. I said to E.R., 'When I meet people I try to find things in them which I respect and admire, things which will help raise my opinion of humanity. But as far as the personal element is concerned, I've no use for them and that gives me a fairly clear judgment, I imagine, and also a great freedom to get on with the job.' That was apparently my philosophy of life at the advanced age of twenty-six! I also loathed and detested the power of money.

I had to find fresh lodgings, which was difficult, but Fannie Wood, who had taught me singing, had a flat at 46 Park Road, Clarence Gate, which she shared with a young German girl and she nobly took me in for very small remuneration. She was kindness itself and a beautiful cook. Local Sussex gossip reported that I was half-starving while studying in London. As a matter of fact I never starved but I did, when I was alone, organise my meals on a system. Quite often I had a meal out at Aunt Betty's or the Yates Thompsons', and the day before, and possibly after, I ate frugally. If on the other hand I went for a week or two with no free meals, I would eat sparingly for three or four meals at little cost and then spend quite a lot on a square meal which I chose with equal care and greed, which meant that I thoroughly enjoyed my food. However, it was not very often that I was left to fend for myself. Generally Miss Wood was at home and fed me admirably; she always had a good supply of fresh eggs and butter from her father's farm. She was often away for weekends, when I had to shop and cook for myself.

I seldom enjoyed Sundays in London but there was one occasion when I had worked myself to a standstill and I rang up Pam [Kettle] at her Medical School flat and caught her in. Pam was a real standby – she was tall, dark, with a big mouth and big hands and had large, brown, sorrowful, rather inscrutable eyes. She was a great feminist, had read everything, admired Ibsen immensely, had a strong sense of humour and a first-class brain. Her judgment on medical matters was flawless and her assessment of personalities was uncanny. 'Come and row in Regent's Park?' I suggested. She jumped at the idea – would take a taxi at once. She was fed up with working for her July examination, fed up with a brother's love affair – he would talk about it to her at every opportunity. We made a bargain as we rowed in our little boat; she was to come again next day and ask me Chemistry questions, and once my examination was over I'd ask her questions – she was a year ahead of me – before her examination. She was a staunch ally, and we discussed many things.

In June 1914 I took Matriculation and failed yet again. Miss Laycock was very firm that I was up to the standard in Chemistry and Botany and couldn't understand how I had managed to fail. Other coaches said I'd good brains but was dreadfully impatient. I was told I hadn't a scientific turn of mind but that didn't matter as I'd a more valuable kind of mind which would see me through all right. I felt between the devil and the deep sea. Friends were particularly kind just then and I was invited to Oving for a weekend, which I greatly enjoyed and felt myself made comfortable in Mrs Yates Thompson's presence, wrapped round by the protecting affection she seemed to emanate.

In August 1914 I went to stay with Aunt Betty and Kite at a Hotel in Cooden Beach. We could think of nothing but the likelihood of war. The news of [the British] ultimatum [to Germany] came almost as a relief. We had kept our word as a nation and people talked of the whole thing being over by Christmas. Kite and I on the golf course saw one of the drafts of the British Expeditionary Force go by in a crowded train for embarkation. The soldiers leant out of the windows and cheered; they seemed very young, and happy to be going to fight for England's honour. We waved back to give them our good wishes, but we were both deeply moved and chokey, however great our admiration for their courage.

I had, once again, to change my lodgings. After long searching, made none the easier by war conditions, I was accepted, through the kind offices of Mrs Yates Thompson, at St George's House, Vincent Square. This was a hostel started by her sister, Miss Ethel Murray Smith, for professional women, secretaries, almoners, and such-like. I was lucky to get a room there. It was small with a shilling in the slot gas-meter stove and ring, and the charges were about thirty shillings weekly for breakfast and supper, Monday to Saturday. Lentil soup was a great standby and how tired I got of it! If you stayed over the weekend you paid more. It was very clean and most of the inmates were nice and kindly disposed. There was only one small silence room where one could sit and study and I did most of my work in my room – secure, I hoped, against inter- ruptions. During all those war years and indeed till I began to keep my own cows, Mrs Yates Thompson sent half to a pound of butter each to E.R. and me weekly. It was an imaginatively kind and generous gift.

Just before the outbreak of war E.R. was being strenuously active over Votes for Women, and Lord and Lady Buxton, as they then were, were waiting for final arrangements about the liner to take them to his job as Governor-General of South Africa. I again became greatly concerned as to the possibility of a breach in the friendship between E.R. and Mildred Buxton. The feelings of both as regards Women's Suffrage ran high on opposing sides, not mitigated by the fact that Lady Sybil Smith (Mildred Buxton's sister-in-law) had been sent to prison for the Cause. I wrote anxiously to E.R. [describing a visit to the Buxtons at Newtimber]:

Says Lady Buxton, reaching out and holding my hot hand for a long while, 'Before you become a militant Suffragette and shoot anybody, I want to give you a book to read. Everything, my dear Tate, is due to Mrs Pankhurst.' I looked affectionately at her, and said I hadn't it in my mind to shoot anyone. But she's worried about me, thinks I'm a brand to be snatched from the burning! Had told Phyllis that I am becoming a militant but Phyllis said it was all much deeper than that.

I was thoroughly worried. I couldn't bear to think of Lady Buxton's going off to South Africa with a sore heart over E.R. Phyllis said how much her mother loved E.R. [despite their disagreements]. Yet Lady Buxton thought all suffragettes were obsessed and could talk of nothing else; she used to be so puzzled that E.R. made that theory nonsense. So I boldly wrote to E.R.: 'That's why I want you to take her by surprise again next time and ignore the subject.' This was the second time I had plunged in to prevent a breach. E.R. and Lady Buxton did not argue next time, they were staunch friends.

I went back to the School of Medicine in my usual depressed frame of mind, meeting all my co-students who were anxious to sympathise, and the teachers, who were chafed at my having to be treated specially over pre-medical subjects until I had mastered Matriculation. Failure in June, failure in September, would I ever pass? I began to wonder. In the end Miss Laycock and others advocated the Cambridge Senior Higher Local, the Mathematics for that examination being much more coachable. But it would mean I could not take the coveted London degree, and should have to be content with the College of Physicians and Surgeons diploma. There was one great advantage in taking this examination; if I failed in some subjects and passed in others I could take it again only in the subjects I had failed. The examination was in December and specified books were set. Over the English I had a great ally in E.R. Parts of *Kenilworth*, *The Tempest*, Browning, John Morley and Meredith were read to me and I was coached in them by E.R. I was allowed to stay at Backset for odd weekends before the ordeal.

The result was that I passed fairly easily in all except Latin, but I could take that separately in three months. What a relief!

To celebrate my success I was allowed, on my birthday in January 1915, to accompany E.R. to Liverpool. She was sailing to the United States of America, but owing to war conditions she had to stay the night at Liverpool. It was with a heavy heart I saw her off, for ships were being torpedoed, and though the United States had not yet joined the Allies, one never felt sure whether the U-boats could always be relied on to discriminate. E.R. returned in March 1915 and I met her at Euston. She was astonished at Henfield's wartime activities. For instance, dashing in the darkness to catch the post she was stopped by a sentinel saying, 'Halt', in fierce tones. She answered truculently, annoyed at being hindered, at which the local inhabitant recognised her voice and said meekly, 'Good evening Miss!' But that wasn't all; she had to register as an alien, and report her movements to the police, and get permits 'to go places'. One of E.R.'s jobs was to lecture to children and others for the Food Ministry.

Before my examination in Latin I went down to Brighton for a week or two of extra coaching from my old friend Miss Lowenstein. Her encouragement gave me the necessary extra confidence and I passed easily. So all the doors were now open wide. I met E.R. in Brighton and we celebrated over a tea at Barbellions!

6

A WOMAN MEDICAL
STUDENT IN WARTIME
1915–18

My success left me feeling on top of the world but a week or so later I had a letter from Mr Nettleton who had been invoked to get me through Physics. He thought it would take a year – i.e. March *1916*. It was most disheartening and he had no idea of my abysmal Mathematics weakness – and Physics needs fundamentally good Mathematics! This was staggering. I suspected that if I worked hard right through the summer my brain would get dried up and incapable of assimilating facts, for I was still handicapped then by a brain which suddenly turned stale. I decided not to abandon the idea of a December examination until I had met him, and he had seen something of my work. He had been frank about terms and warned me of the expense of private coaching. I had by this time come to the wise decision that I would try for no more examinations on the outside chance. I must feel thoroughly equipped.

I decided to carry on at St George's House in spite of the long trek to Hunter Street. The hostel was comfortably near Aunt Betty, Uncle Basil and Victoria Station. Moreover, though I was interested in other people's lives I did not relish being absorbed in a wholly student atmosphere. I preferred a mixed bag of acquaintances who were none of them likely to interfere with my liberty. It was a friendly atmosphere of women of different ages in many different walks of life. Perhaps because I was shy I found it comfortably impersonal.

It was possible to have a couple of visitors to supper so long as one gave the staff notice. This I did on one occasion when my guests, who had invited themselves, were two students of my year. They stayed long and late and I began to wonder how

I could best turn them out. One was tall and dark with large, melancholy brown eyes which she fixed upon me in a way that made me feel uncomfortable. I found that their individual outlook, their background and their philosophy were totally different from mine. But they were well educated and well read. A day or two later they sent me flowers and asked me to supper in return. I made the excuse of being too busy, and refused.

Then the tall one began to wait and wanted to take me to my bus, to accompany me home. I took a violent dislike to her and tried to evade her, but she was worse than Mary's little lamb in her persistent following of my footsteps. She began to haunt St George's House and she got on my nerves. I would leave instructions that I was out. She sent me presents of jewellery which I gave back to the school porter who took them with a sympathetic grin and promised to deliver the parcel to her. My room at St George's House was on the first floor and had a transom so that anybody down the passage could see if my light was on, and she would often wait outside in the street. When I appeared, intent on dining with Aunt Betty, she would suddenly emerge from a doorway, seize me by the arm, and try to coerce me to accompany her. I grew terrified of her. I did not know how to shake her off. I told her I was busy, I had not a moment to spare and would she leave me alone. She laughed and thought I was joking. I finally went to the Dean of the Medical School who was sympathetic but doubted if she could put a stop to her pestering me; besides the girl was well connected and she did not want to antagonise her parents. Occasionally, she reassured me, there were queer girls who behaved like that but they got over it. I was very disturbed and my work suffered until two kind sisters who were secretaries at St George's sensed I was being pestered; they offered their room for me to study in and my own room was left in darkness. I wrote to consult E.R. but she thought I must have been encouraging the girl.

When I had travelled to Liverpool with E.R., before she sailed to New York, I had asked if she would allow me to look upon her as my adopted mother. She had agreed to this and had said that I might call her Monna. This I did in letters but hardly ever in speech. I did not connect it, in my dimness, with Monna Lisa (Lady Bell and all her friends called her Lisa), nor did I know that she consciously shied from anything in the nature of a mother complex.

I use the term 'dimness' because at that period I was completely ignorant of one side of behaviour. I had accepted the fact that many girls had devoted friendships, which were both normal and healthy, as in fact I had with Joan and Phyllis. But this obsession on the part of X.Y., as I will call her, suddenly struck me as something ugly, alarming, unhinged. What did it mean? I was twenty-eight years old and considered myself well versed in the ways of the world. I knew about the work of Josephine Butler who had devoted her energies to the moral elevation, protection and reclamation of women from the dangers of prostitution. Dr Martindale's *Under the Surface* and E.R.'s *Where Are You Going To* had further indoctrinated me [about the evils of the White Slave Traffic]. I was familiar with the problems of illegitimacy, abortion and 'living in sin', though I never remember such matters being topics of conversation in ordinary society, nor even among the medical students of my day. But of homosexuality I knew nothing. It is not surprising that X.Y.'s behaviour, and the guarded explanations of what I had taken to be mental derangement, came as a considerable shock to my innocence. I was thankful that at St George's House I was further away from her potential clutches, but she became a consuming problem to me. Fortunately the second wind I gained over passing examinations, the distractions of wartime conditions, and above all the harrying of my teachers, did finally eliminate the incident from my mind.

One summer's day I was asked to accompany the Dean of the Medical School, Miss Aldrich-Blake, down to Rolls Park where Lady Sybil Smith was having a meeting at which the Dean was to speak. Miss Aldrich-Blake was a tall, massive individual who wore a stiff collar and a tie like a man's. She was later made a Dame for her admirable surgery. Sybil Smith looked upon her as the 'sheep in wolf's clothing', as she was sure she was a man. I described the trip in a letter to E.R.:

It's suddenly become a furnace, terribly hot. Tonight is
the night that, from all sides, one hears we are to have
Zeppelins again. A man in the War Office told Pam Kettle's
brother. The last lot dropped papers on the coast saying they
were to be expected again today, and it's true that I've never
seen London so empty all in a moment.

Yesterday was entertaining, and I'm quite intrigued as
regards Miss Aldrich-Blake. I sat next to her going down and
coming back from Rolls. There were also two others, Miss
Brooks, and Mrs G. The bulk of the conversation was carried
on by Mrs G. She insisted on sitting with her back to the
driver; Miss Aldrich-Blake, ponderously polite, lifted her and
the seat to a better angle, even though Mrs G protested
that she was most comfortable. And ten minutes later Miss
Aldrich-Blake insisted upon Mrs G's moving to a different
corner.

'Now I see where your wonderful success lies; it's because
you always compel people to do what you want in spite of
all protests,' says Mrs G to Miss Aldrich-Blake. *Beams* on
the part of the latter, who never opened lips unless one
metaphorically poked her in the ribs.

'Oh, but don't you think that it's part of the equipment
of a woman doctor to be an out and out autocrat?' I asked.
Miss Aldrich-Blake grunted approval and beamed again.

'Yes, I suppose it is. You see, all women love power and
usually they have to get it by mean ways, but as a doctor
you can be quite open and honest in your commanding.'

My object was to get into touch with Miss Aldrich-Blake.
One wants to put things very clearly, no frills, no hidden
meaning, no jokes. And then one does it as one talks to a
very young child. Then, she'll perhaps get there and respond.
I like her. Good all through, imperturbable equanimity,
nerves of iron for operating, I'm sure. But speechless. I
should feel every confidence in her slicing one into bits deliberately and never losing her head at any crisis. I'd like awfully
to see something of her as it would give me more pleasure
than I can say to stir her up somehow, to some enthusiasm
or emotion. But I don't believe it would be possible!

75

[At Rolls Park] last of all spoke Miss Aldrich-Blake, not a speaker, but looking a perfect rock of good nature and serenity. Two things won my respect. Very frankly and honestly, with no idea of doing it well, she dropped out quite simply that a surgeon's life was the happiest in the world. And she *looked* like it. And nothing is healthy in the world unless it shows growth. It's true, isn't it? She has a gift of peaceful calm, and sitting next to her one literally felt she radiated strength. I always get feelings of some kind from my next neighbour, as to their predominant characteristics, and after sitting next to any one I have quite decided intuitions about them. I'm not sure that this kind of sensitiveness mayn't be very valuable to me later on.

With the sinking of the *Lusitania* on 7 May 1915 I became war haunted. I tried to shake off my dejection by going out to Wimbledon with three other students to get fresh air, but I only felt more tired. So I rang up Pam [Kettle] and asked her to go with me to hear Uncle Basil preach about the *Lusitania* as it would be 'hot stuff'. She came, and though an agnostic, was impressed by his language, logic and personality. The church was packed and numbers of khaki-clad men were there; before the war women had predominated. I had a word with Uncle Basil afterwards. He talked of E.R., of my mother, of my work. He was immensely interested in obstetrics and said he would give me a lot of tips as to how, by manipulation alone, great alleviation could be effected! He had unexpectedly wide knowledge of medical matters. He talked about my affairs and said he had quarrelled with my mother about me. They thought it derogatory that I should want to take up a profession, but he had maintained it was everything praiseworthy. He asked how much money they allowed me and was horrified at the answer. He was very sympathetic, encouraging and kind, and told me always to come to him when I felt depressed.

E.R. and Beatrice Harraden were acting as librarians in the Endell Street Military Hospital, which was staffed entirely by medical women, as the War Office had ruled that they should not be sent abroad. Dr Flora Murray and Miss Louisa Garrett

Anderson were the officers in charge and E.R. took many friends and journalists over the hospital. These included J.L. Garvin of the *Observer* and Horatio Bottomley of *John Bull*.

'But who operates when seriously wounded casualties are drafted in?' asked these innocents.

They were gently and firmly told, 'The women surgeons, naturally,' and E.R. would turn them loose in the wards to talk privately to the soldiers. She chuckled afterwards at their warm enthusiasm when they rejoined her later, greatly enlightened and converted to the work of medical women.

I decided I would have a shot at the Biology examination in July 1915 and was invited to Backset for the last ten pre-examination days. This put me into good heart and on 24 July I heard I had passed the Biology examination.

That autumn the Medical School was opened by HM Queen Mary. It was a great occasion for us. Queen Mary insisted on seeing everything, even the dissecting room, which for a lay person was, I should have thought, something of an ordeal. Apart from the sights, the smell of formaldehyde, combined with the mummified parts of the human body, made a most unwelcoming stench. According to plan she was being hurried through as rapidly as possible, but Her Majesty's enquiring eye was not to be fobbed off with a superficial glance. She firmly stopped at Pam's bench and, peering into a peculiarly unpleasant mess of guts: 'And what, may I ask, is that section you are working on?'

Pam quickly rallied to the Majestic occasion, felt it would be indelicate to answer 'Guts', and said smilingly, 'This Ma'am, is the material we have to work with to learn Anatomy' – and with her accustomed dignity, Queen Mary thanked her and moved on.

The air was full of rumours about Gallipoli and the leadership of Sir Ian Hamilton, E.R.'s friend. Our war policy was criticised sharply in the accustomed British way, and anxiety was rife as to possibly continuous Zeppelin raids. We had already had a few, leaving a certain amount of damage in their wake.

Joan Campion suddenly became engaged and was married in December 1915 in London, just before my Physics and Chemistry examination. She looked radiantly lovely, while he looked old enough to be her father. I felt desperately miserable. Joan was a nervous, shy person, but she rose to the occasion and was tactful and gentle and behaved perfectly. I met her fiancé, Heber Pack, and wrote doubtfully to E.R.:

> Was it very uncivil not to say polite things to old Pack? The epithet fits metaphorically in my mind, so forgive it. He says 'Thankee' and 'Lookee, there's a stir!' Just so long as *I* don't marry him I expect it will be right. My experience (limited!) of men who have that soapy soothing voice is that they have devilish tempers underneath.

The whole thing was apparently nearly broken off because he would not provide for his daughters in the settlement. The Campions, gentlemanly and honest, had to exert pressure and he was forced to give in.

The subsequent history proved revealing. Joan, whose chief enjoyment was to play the piano up to four hours a day, was not allowed to do so as her husband didn't like the noise. This also applied to their child. After endless beseeching, her husband finally allowed her to put up double doors, and playing the piano and playing with Tommie were carried on in peaceful banishment. Joan was not happy but she was very reserved and had great powers of endurance; only once did she ever admit to her sister Mary anything of what she had to put up with for about eighteen years. Her husband had three characteristics developed to the utmost: meanness (he was very rich), jealousy and cruelty. When he died, Joan benefited by his will to the extent of a silver teapot. Nothing more! She later married Commander Archie Domvile, and was divinely happy in his quiet devotion and the social life that he gave her.

Meanwhile I was busy working for the Physics and Chemistry examination. Miss Laycock was keeping a watchful eye over my Chemistry. I could not absorb Physics which was too much based on mathematical knowledge. Miss Laycock had settled that at the Birkbeck College I was to have private coaching from Mr (later Professor) H.R. Nettleton. He was a grave, sallow rather owlish-looking man with a genius for cramming and a great gift for making clear the intricacies of Physics. I had to go in the evenings, which have never been the best hours for my brain, and I was tired after the day's work at school. As regards my chances in the examination he thought it would depend on the questions. He said I knew certain things very well and could pass comfortably on those, but I might strike subjects where I would be altogether at sea. He gave me confidence by his frank assessment.

The 1915 Christmas holiday was spent at Bramlands. Once again I was subjected to every kind of abuse about my behaviour in not staying at home to look after my mother and the absurdity of my imagining that with my lack of brains I could ever pass examinations. I went over to E.R. as often as possible as an antidote and she invited me for the long weekend immediately before the examination. She read me chapters of her half-finished novel *Camilla* and I was thrilled by it, and, as she read the chapters about Florida, out of the ashes of the wood fire there crept a small lizard! Never before had there been such a visitor. We were enchanted and took it as a good omen. I left Backset soothed and encouraged, and wrote to tell her that I did not agree with the theory that good work is done only by the unhappy; for examinations one had to be feeling on top of things. In the strain of examination times, it made all the difference to know that someone took an affectionate interest in the result. Mr Nettleton was the other person who helped a lot; he cared as a sculptor cares for the clay he has moulded. On 6 January 1916 I wrote to E.R.:

The practical Physics is over. I had to find the volume of a glass rod by displacement of water. And I did it wrong. Never done experiment before! Wasn't it awful? I couldn't remember theoretically how it was done. Along came examiner and I told him the result. He asked me what I meant by a certain statement. I told him.

'Then why did you put that?' Now, the whole of the examination depended on my answer. I'd seen this little man with florid face, about fifty-five, bullying to the last degree.

And I thought my only chance was to get on what might be his best side (I'd heard one person excuse himself by saying he was nervous and the examiner was made furious by it), so I said with the utmost withering self-contempt 'Simply idiotic of me'.

Says he, 'You have yourself supplied the adjective. *Now* see whether you can rectify the rest.' And he departed. I rectified it, and found the area again too. Then being frantically anxious I found the area of the beastly thing another way (because when he first came to see whether I'd done it right he checked it this other way on a little card). So when he came round again I very humbly and meekly say, 'I've got it to .23 sq. cms. And I've confirmed it by measuring the diameter and saying area – MR square'.

'Did you?' said he with a good deal of astonishment, evidently impressed.

He led me to a table strewn with apparatus: 'Do you know what any of these are for?' and he began by touching a galvanometer. I knew that. Another thing. Hygrometer. All right. Spherometer, all right. But I'd seen it only once in a picture. Fearful luck to remember its silly name. 'Well, that will do.' And he took my arm, squeezed it and led me to the door. I thanked him warmly. There was an air of finality about him as if he didn't expect to see me again in three months. I may be unduly hopeful. But some people say that if you right yourself from a bad experiment they give you greater credit than if you get it right straight away. Some of the others were being perfect fools, and that always encourages me.

The results came through – I had passed. I went to thank Mr Nettleton and told him everything. He questioned me closely.

'And you had only been shown that once and you remembered?' He blinked at me with a mixture of gratified pleasure and surprise. We parted the best of friends.

In February 1917 I was still at Vincent Square, struggling with Physiology, which I enjoyed, and Anatomy, which became a nightmare. There was so much pure memory required. It needed a trained mind to memorise pure facts. I had a good memory for facts which had a reason for them, and physiological and particularly medical data I absorbed by osmosis. But the Anatomy examinations loomed menacingly. I enjoyed dissection, though the detailed picking out of nerves and vessels was a more than lengthy proceeding. A limb of the human body was shared by two students and it took us all our skill to do this adequately in the time at our disposal. Without the painstaking help and inspired teaching of Mrs Mary Lucas Keene (now Professor Emeritus in Anatomy, University of London, a distinction never before awarded to a woman), I doubt if I should ever have passed my Anatomy examination. After I had failed I had private coaching from her, and her patience, as I look back, must have far outrivalled that of Job.

She strongly advised me not to attempt the next Anatomy examination in June 1917 but to put it off for three months; my knowledge was not up to the required standard. This was a great blow. I was thirsting to get on to real patients, and away from dull facts of memory and specimens. Again I developed my usual cowardice and became gloomy and dejected. Whenever I went home to Bramlands I had to endure the usual discouragement and was firmly told I could never hope to get through. It was the duty of every girl to have a baby in order to help the war effort, my sister Barbara added!

In spite of Mrs Lucas Keene's advice I took the Anatomy examination again in June. I thought the experience would help me and I obstinately had a shot at it, only to fail! In September I tackled it again. There were fairly frequent air raids all that autumn, and police in the streets suddenly displayed large placards 'take cover'. On 1 October I planned to take E.R. to Queen Square, the examination hall where the results were posted. We tried to get a taxi, but there was another raid and it was impossible. We couldn't get there and were left in suspense. The next day there was yet another raid, [but we eventually discovered that] I'd passed! I was finished with Anatomy and Physiology and on an impulse we went along to Westminster Abbey and told the news to William Wilberforce sitting benignly in his marble chair.

I had already begun impatiently to plan ahead in talks with Pam Kettle. When she had passed her Physiology and Anatomy well ahead of me, the question of where to take the clinical work had to be decided. Instead of automatically going to the Royal Free, at that time the only hospital in London open to women students, she considered the alternative possibility of St Mary's Hospital, Paddington. St Mary's was hard up for students' fees, as the war had absorbed nearly all the available young men, and the hospital was willing to accept a few women as an experiment. The School of Medicine were loath to see Pam and her set go to St Mary's Hospital, but Pam was a strong personality, much respected by the staff, and a natural leader of enterprise. It mattered enormously that the women allowed to invade such a malebound, prejudiced hospital, where Sir Almroth Wright was looked up to as a god, should be a carefully chosen band who could be relied on to make a good impression. We talked endlessly and she gave me her views of the teaching staff at St Mary's Hospital. When I was through the second medical she'd like me to join them at St Mary's Hospital and thought I'd do well in that free air of coeducation. She asked me over and took me round the wards and even the smell of the place attracted me. Porters, sisters, nurses all seemed to treat my friend with warm welcoming courtesy. There was not a sign of antagonism, even in the nursing staff; there was less work for nurses as they did not have to chaperon when women patients were examined.

I began my work in St Mary's Hospital, Paddington, as a dresser in Casualty in October 1917. It was a sound method to throw the raw beginner into the deep end. Severely injured, bleeding, sometimes unconscious, patients of all ages were brought in from the north side of Hyde Park. Many were brought in by the police, whom I quickly learned were among the kindest of men. Some were drunks and quite violent, and there was an occasional malingerer who feigned fits in order to gain a bed for a night. The Casualty Sister was elderly, Irish, and stood no nonsense. As dressers you had to do exactly as she ordered after the Casualty House Surgeon had diagnosed and dictated treatment. She chivied us all mercilessly and insisted on our being really helpful to the patients, whatever their plight. One learned a good deal about London night life on Casualty. My first days, when I was clad in a new white coat, and feeling very professional, were eye-opening to the last degree and frankly horrified me by the bloody sights and sounds of mankind literally in the raw, hurt and moaning and afraid. The House Surgeon I worked for was an Irishman with a nice voice, and a civil manner, very gentle in his handling of patients. If he was not too rushed he would explain his methods and answer my eager questions.

The 'firms' I was allocated to work with were carefully selected by Pam, who was a couple of years ahead and knew all the ropes. (A firm comprised the Surgeon and House Surgeon with surgical dressers in attendance, or the Physician and House Physician with clinical clerks in attendance. In effect we, as dressers or clerks, were learners.) Loyalty to one's chief was fierce. If a surgeon cursed and swore or threw an unsuitable instrument on the floor of the operating theatre, didn't it add spice to life? By and large it was the surgeons who were the most sarcastic and fierce, not only with students, but even with patients who were sometimes malingerers. The physicians had a gentler, subtler approach. I was responsible for 'my' patients (especially when the air raid sirens went). Every student was given so many patients to take histories from and diagnose ready for the chief's round, so one naturally accepted responsibility, reassured the nervous ones and bluffed with such imper- turbability that we calmed ourselves as well as the patients.

What thrilled and absorbed my interest was when my turn came to be a clinical clerk. Pam advised me to put my name down for Dr Wilfred Harris: 'Not only will you find him a first rate teacher, but you'll work in Alexandra and Albert Wards. Sister Albert (Amy Fooks) on the men's wards will teach you more medicine than anybody in the hospital. She is a byword for her clinical observation but a great tartar. Will stand no nonsense, so get on her right side.' I learned that probationers would tremble in their shoes and come out white- faced and scared after their first days in Albert or Cambridge ward under this martinet. 'That girl who has come out top in her examinations is conceited and useless, doesn't even know how to make a patient's pillows comfortable, and as to giving bed pans, I don't know if I can ever lick her into shape,' Sister Albert would say despairingly. She was relentless in her efforts, none the less. At the end of two or three weeks the girl would either go to Matron in tears to ask for a transfer or would tell all her friends she was unspeakably grateful for being in Albert under its dreaded but esteemed disciplinarian teacher.

All the medical chiefs sought Sister Albert's clinical help in both diagnosis and prognosis, including Dr Sidney Phillips, whom she hero-worshipped. Dr Phillips was a great doctor, remarkable for his clinical observation and acumen. When he gave a tutorial he might glance down the line of beds, see a man who gave a short cough and was lying in a particular position, and say, 'Got a case of pleurisy haven't you, Sister, in No. 6?'

'That's what I thought, Sir, but he has only just come in and hasn't been examined yet' – she'd beam reverently in reply. And we'd all gasp at this clinical observation and be thrilled when the lightning diagnosis was confirmed after extensive examination. I did my best to cultivate Sister Albert and in the end she became my dearest friend in hospital. She put the welfare of her patients before every other consideration in life.

Meanwhile in the women's ward I had a stroke of luck over a patient who had been sent in for diagnosis and was a puzzle. Reading over my examination notes, where I had said she couldn't differentiate in her arms between the sensations of heat and cold, Dr Harris gave me a quick look and sent for test tubes of hot and cold water and went over her in his meticulously careful way. He looked at me again, and before the whole class said, 'A brilliant piece of observation – this is a case of syringomyelia which had not been diagnosed,' and went on with a long illuminating description of this complaint. I was utterly flabbergasted and flushed.

'Don't forget,' he ended, 'you can never know in medicine what you may not learn from an observant and inexperienced student.' He would constantly say to us: 'More things are missed by not looking than by not knowing', and 'When a patient is sent to you with a ready made diagnosis always assume it's wrong till you've made up your own mind'. I was blissfully happy in my clinical work and astonished by the post mortems. Dr Bernard Spilsbury or Dr Kettle used to do them with all the speed and efficiency of great craftsmen. It looked misleadingly simple, as I was to realise later to my never-to-be-forgotten dismay.

My time at St Mary's was one of the happiest periods of my life. I was working hard and learning all the time what I wanted to learn and not just trying to assimilate facts, as a means to an end. I was also absorbing a great deal of knowledge about people of every class, age and occupation. The war was still on and there was the unforgettable spirit of striving together against the common enemy and, however inconvenient things might be, we all struggled together in a bond of amity. I was also taught manners. Being a ridiculously shy person I would try to slip into the hospital as far as possible unnoticed and with no greeting, but the admirable porters, who never forgot a name or a face, would always intercept me, 'Good morning Miss Wilberforce', and I realised that it was expected of me to reply 'Good morning'. It seems a small thing, but I'd never been told that it mattered, so hadn't previously bothered. In every hospital there must always be a spirit of goodwill and reassurance pervading the place, of a united wish to help against the enemies, disease and death. This was magnified in time of war, though there were inevitably some rivalries and much competition.

The autumn of 1917 had found E.R. constantly ill which was a great anxiety for me. Part of the time she was at Backset with very uncertain domestic help and then a good deal at a friend's home in St Leonard's Terrace, Chelsea. I stole time to get away and fill hot water bottles and cook her delicacies which she had to be persuaded to eat. I had been living at St George's House and growing more than ever intolerant of the monotonous food. In early December we booked three rooms at three and a half guineas a week at 6 Cambridge Terrace for both E.R. and myself. It would be very handy for St Mary's and I could keep an eye on her health. Two Devonian sisters, Mrs Ward and

Miss Snell, ran the place and were excellent cooks, and I did the shopping. They were a kind and patient couple for my hours were unpredictable owing to the need for emergency operations and so on, and E.R. might be delayed by air raids at any of her Food Ministry talks. I think they were fascinated by her visitors, the Ian Hamiltons, Somerset Maugham, Hugh Walpole and the Hugh Bells, among others.

Number 6 Cambridge Terrace was not a luxury establishment, but we had a pleasant sun-filled sitting-room on the first floor, rather over-full of heavy Victorian furniture, and two bedrooms on the second floor. The bedrooms both had old-fashioned iron double beds which took up almost the whole room, but they were quite reasonably comfortable. When air raids came along we all descended to the stone staircase in the basement. On a few occasions after emergency operations at the hospital I was so tired I begged to be allowed to sleep in my bed – guns or no guns. It is surprising how inured one can become to almost any sort of noise if sufficiently sleepy. After a time I became so much interested in my ward work at St Mary's that I would sleep through the sirens and distant gunfire. E.R. would softly open the door, find me sound asleep, and go back to her own room, not thinking it worthwhile to go down below, unless the noise of the guns came nearer. It only took me about ten minutes to walk to hospital, so I often dashed back to lunch in the earlier days as I felt shy in the Common Room at St Mary's. Women were in a minority among the students and were tolerated rather than welcomed, and being a good bit older than the average student, I probably felt doubly ill at ease and diffident.

The news that Denis Buxton was killed was the greatest shock of the war. I remembered how, when he was eighteen, his uncles had agitated that he should be his father's ADC or go on the staff in British East Africa, both comparatively safe jobs. Sydney Buxton had already lost two sons, but the boy and his immediate family saw only one course of duty to be followed. I think he did the right thing. I wrote to E.R.:

Now these poor Buxtons will feel that if they had insisted

on his serving [in East Africa] things might be different. I personally have never known any boy so closely as I've known Denis, and I can't imagine it possible for anybody to be created who was so lovable or more faithfully affectionate. Weeping, bicycling across the Park, I became aware that was why a sentry, and other people, stared at me! Idiotic lack of self control.

I wished I had been in London and had seen him the last time he was home. He always was kind enough to want to see me, and I bear a grudge against my examinations now to think they sometimes intervened.

When the maroons sounded for the Armistice on the morning of 11 November 1918 we were given the day off and I tore from the hospital, not bothering to collect my hat. I ran down Cambridge Terrace with tears streaming down my face at the thought of Denis Buxton's sacrifice. Why couldn't he, of all the promising youth I knew, have been spared? E.R. had heard the maroons and thought they were an air raid warning in answer to Armistice terms; but Mrs Ward had gone in exclaiming, 'Peace, Peace', and they had embraced. E.R. went on to the balcony and saw me tearing down the street. We seized our coats, and went out into the street. She bought a Union Jack and I a Stars and Stripes flag and we hailed a taxi to Buckingham Palace where already there was a sea of people cheering and waving flags. The big gates were thrown open and the sentry was smiling as United States' soldiers and sailors with a huge United States' flag carried it into the yard. The noise of the cheering was terrific and we were nearly crushed against the tall railings.

7
MIDWIFERY IN DUBLIN
1918

In July 1918, accompanied by a student from the Royal Free
Hospital, called Bellows, I went to do my practical midwifery
at the Rotunda Hospital in Dublin, which claimed to be the
best in the world at that time. The period at the Rotunda was
an eye-opening experience. I had never been in Ireland before.
I remembered nothing of the voyage over, except that I was
mildly seasick and thankful to arrive. The Rotunda was a queer-
looking building, not at all one's idea of a hospital, but it was
admirably run, spotlessly clean and the food was superb. I've
always had a keen appreciation – in other words been greedy
– of good food. It was in itself an immense treat to have bacon,
ham, butter, sugar – all free and plentiful after the difficulties
of English rationing. The bathroom, with unlimited hot water,
was huge and this was more than a luxury. The weather was
very hot.

Messages would come and, after suitable briefing, the student
was sent out armed with a precious 'midder' bag to a case in
some street reached partly by tram, partly on foot. Occasionally, the husband would come up with a verbal message
and that made it easier as he would guide one back. My first
few visits were rather alarming but I soon came to love the Irish
as patients. I entered a dark bedroom, often on the ground
floor, where the patient was being tended by relatives or neighbours, all supported with strong cups of tea. She would be
groaning with pains. I would put down my bag, ask for kettles
of hot water to be put on the old-fashioned coal stove, and take
the patient's hand and feel her pulse and abdomen. In two
minutes the tears and the groans would cease and she'd feel

quite reassured. I'd quickly put on my sterile gown, proceed to wash her, don my sterilised rubber gloves after careful washing of my hands and arms, if there was time and enough water available, before I examined her internally. This was the period when Lloyd George had instituted a thirty-shilling maternity benefit to help prepare for the confinement and provide adequate clothing for the baby, but the Irish had their own special preferences as to the outlay of the thirty shillings. Sometimes it was whisky, but often it was a beautiful ham that was boiling away cheerfully and taking up all the available space on the stove. It took considerable persuasion to convince the relatives that kettles of boiling water were to have priority if I were to deal successfully with the delivery. Once the kettle had boiled, the ham would resume its cooking on the grate. Nature is in most cases an efficient obstetrician, and many of my ministrations were of a hygienic, common sense and lessening of pain nature. But not always.

[Octavia Wilberforce's Dublin midwifery experience is described through her vivid letters to Elizabeth Robins:]

July 14 1918   Rotunda Hospital   Dublin
Best and most beloved of all the Monnas in the world,
   We were shown rooms (Bellows had gathered from the syllabus we might have to share one, so I was greatly relieved – simply couldn't have borne it), fairly nice rooms as regards size and bed. Bath clean and hot, day or night, tho' ceilings and walls black to a degree! From what I've seen there's every likelihood of having heaps of work – one goes alone to a case, after first having done two in hospital, where you have nurses and a sister to help and direct. But they say it's most interesting and the only drawback is fleas, hundreds and thousands of 'em. I'm to buy Keatings [flea powder].
   I've just been idiotic and had to come away from an internal measurements under anaesthetic because – forsooth! I felt faint. Perfectly infantile and childish. Just tired I suppose. Restless night last night, the very noisiest place you can imagine – sounds like dropping bombs or upsetting milkcans

the whole night thro' – maybe one will grow accustomed to that however. Your photograph guards the dressing table.

They've stopped patients having visitors owing to influenza; they stand *no* nonsense here in the interests of health!

I'm most desperately homesick and feel terribly losted [sic] without you to come to with my adventures. I simply implore you to write fairly often. However brief, just the sight of beloved writing will make all the difference to my days.

Your most loving
Sussex Child

July 15
Own darling Monna,

Nothing of interest to report. Round and lecture with Jellett [the Master] this morning and after that, gynaecological exams with him. He's a nice man with an Irish accent and as autocratic as never was. There is a fiery notice forbidding flatly any of the staff or students to go to plays, cinemas or inside trams because of 'flu. Quick, glib, hot tempered with a keen humour. He just manages every smallest detail himself and stands no nonsense from anybody. He's undeniably first-rate and that's the main thing, isn't it? Breezy and healthy minded and above all keen. Stupid students take exception to his manners, but after all he's in authority and, if he's quick and impatient with you, it's all for the purpose of trying to teach you – which he needn't bother to do unless he likes. He puts up notices to say we mustn't be late for meals, unless at a case, and so on. The result is that everybody squirms at the Master's name.

Saw an infant born yesterday. Uncommon simple arrangement when you have a sister rubbing the abdomen, one nurse holding up the mother's leg, another manipulating the child's head and a student dealing with the cord. Please realise *all this* has to be done alone and unaided by me when my turn comes and – worst of everything – the washing up one does in order to be aseptic is so easy in a hospital and so fearfully difficult in their houses, where one has to raise four basins of hot water. However, I'm looking forward to it with much confidence since I'm sure I'm no less intelligent than the average student over these practical details. Perhaps tomorrow evening I may be sent out, it's all luck. I have to get my two cases in the hospital first. You may as well pray that the very first case isn't a primapara – i.e. one who hasn't borne children before.

How I detest continual 'society' – people at breakfast and all meals in great profusion, all chattering incessantly. The noise is so fatiguing. Also, I have to listen so very carefully to understand what all these varieties of Irish accent are saying.

Two Assistant-Masters: One, Dr Gilmour, a disagreeable expressioned Sinn Fein young man, either very conceited or rather shy. I think the former. T'other, Dr Simpson, also young, horrid mouth, pince nez, large black eyes and quite moderately nice to the patients. Is uncommon good at his job, but uncommon conceited too. Chief Clinical Clerk, Dr English: kind, helpful, nice creature. Junior Clinical Clerk, Dr Michael: woman, black, an utter fool over her work from even the little I know. But most willing to try and help. When one is at the case and anything abnormal happens (I shan't know whether it's abnormal or not, probably) one fills up a form which is brought to the Clinical Clerk, and either English or Michael come to the rescue or send a message as to what should be done.

Do write, my darling.

S.C.

6.45 a.m. July 16

Glory be to God for my belovedest, most darling Monna. Here was I getting as impatient as it's possible and longing for word from you and at 6.30 last night happened the first of my internal cases. I dashed upstairs to the labour ward and found the woman with four nurses in attendance, lying groaning and sweating and doing her part. This went on till quarter to eight. Then the child was born. 'Glory be to God it's a boy, Glory be to God it's a boy,' gasped the woman. She was fairly exhausted, it was her first one.

Between you and me, very confidentially, it's all a filthy job. The smell is so disgusting. However, I foresee I shall enjoy it for this reason, that it's a gigantic job single handed and it will need every inch of intelligence and resource to carry thro' decently. One will be immensely keen to save tears of the perineum, which is the distinguishing feature of those who are good at the job.

Beyond all question this was the right place to come to. Good technique, good asepsis, good teaching. Interested (but shocked) to find that Bellows thought it was enough, after using rubber finger stalls, to put them in disinfectant before re-using them. Of course, they must be boiled. I'm glad I'm at St Mary's where they fuss about these details.

Bless you forever,

Your very loving,

S.C.

P.S. I'm covered with huge weals [from flea bites] and the irritation is appalling. It's an awful curse.

July 22 1918

I awoke feeling such a rag this morning – just tired for no reason except that it's a limpyfying place and it's a bit of an effort to do one's round and go visiting the patients who have the misfortune (or otherwise) to belong to me. I think they like me – seem to, but they're all well mannered liars, so one never really knows. You don't realise the utter fatigue of a mad students' life, the chief effect of which is that you only want to be alone to rest yourself, without endless talking.

[Octavia encouraged E.R. to stay at Rounton during Lady Bell's illness, as long as she was needed.] If I don't see you for some weeks after I return from here, it will just mean that each week longer apart will only accentuate and concentrate the nearness when we do come together again, won't it? I mean absence isn't going to make a pin's difference to us now, is it? I don't feel it should at all, just because we have grown so close. I'm more than a daughter and a son and ten children altogether, as far as loving you is concerned,

Monna mine. Will you admit that? Belovedest, ours is a closer relation than has *ever* been welded before.

Do you know what I was thinking yesterday? Bellows said more than anything in the world she'd like to have a baby. I said I didn't want one. Bellows: 'Many girls want children far more than they want a husband.' That seems to me odd, too. I'd certainly put the husband first and then the children, if I had to be landed with one or other. But the truth is this. Since I began Medicine seriously, I've confidently believed that I'm not going to be atrociously bad at it – that some day I may be of quite real use medically. To be anything of a good doctor, if you want to live up to any kind of ideal (women doctors have higher ideals naturally than the common run of men) you'd be no use – or at least never in the higher class – if you were married (lower class doesn't satisfy my ideas); and you'd be never any use with a lot of close ties. You can only concentrate utterly on two things; one, the health of the world, essentially impersonal, and one, essentially personal – my love for you.

Darling, don't you see that it's heaven sent for me to have this relationship? You see, nobody was ever born with such a store, a wealth of caring as your Sussex Child. Consequently, nobody could be more easily lonely if I'd never known you (and therefore more easily worried and career ruined). Since I have you, nobody is more satisfied up to the hilt, more lavished in affection, more continuously pouring at your feet every drop of love in my whole being as this your devoted child. So you see how completely blessed am I. And in consequence what a good doctor I will be. Everything is interwoven, dependent on my caring for you, which is the end and aim of my life.

P.S. Will you answer this letter, my darling? Because it isn't often I let as much affection as this get into a letter.

July 23
I do hope this next case, when it comes, will be a nice proper normal one for me to deal with from beginning to end. Ye Gods! but the poverty – the filth of some rooms.

Today I was very, very nearly sick by the animal condition of a child on the floor – dogs are cleaner, and the poor mother too easily saw the disgust of my face and apologised . . . wasn't it dreadful?

Farewell, dear heart. You're the most blessed Monna ever was to write such beloved letters to your very far away child. Your ever very loving,

S.C.

July 24

They're a damnable set of slackers these people over here. When one walks along any street one meets crowds and crowds of young men, all talking and smoking and spitting. Heaven knows what occupation they have – it's certainly not an arduous one. And then they congregate in groups round the 'Call for men recruiting notices' and underline the word 'Liberty' and cross out or tear off 'God save the king'! It's not military service so much as work I'd like to see 'em at. They're everything that's charming and well mannered and underneath the biggest liars and the greatest slovens the world can produce. It's really rather a pathetic nation, I feel.

I personally am momentarily bored with this job. I've waited three days in vain for a case. Today Bellows had one. Ugh, such a monster. Won't tell you about it – too disgusting. It waved an arm and she was afraid it would live – tried hurriedly to think how she could nefariously kill it (legally you commit murder if you do). The mother-in-law called for water. Bellows panicking that it would be resuscitated – but they only wanted to baptise it hurriedly, 'Theresa'. Mother nearly died, creature did die and was lost by Bellows in the bed! I think babies, and the bearing of children, and the possibility of what haunting hideosities they may prove to be, is altogether one of the beastliest proceedings ever made. For the first time in my life I realise why Providence, when he wanted to curse womankind, did it that way. A newborn infant is always a beastly little thing, horrible smelling and dirty beyond words to look at. Pain is the least evil of it to my thinking, tho' God knows that's bad enough.

If I do night work, it won't be just yet. In any case there'd be not the faintest anxiety attached to it. Because tho' there's a fairly strong anti-English feeling, nobody is going to interfere with a doctor. And for the rest, men are drunk and women fight in the streets just as much in the daytime as at night. Indeed it's far more peaceful at night because all the clubs and meetings have been stopped by the Irish police, so that people have to stay at home, as a man explained to me, from sheer boredom!

I'm overdone with the infants. How an otherwise fairly sane creature like Maude Royden could sentimentalise over this work fairly amazes me. The one refreshing thing is the way Assistant Masters, students all ages and sexes, and qualified doctors talk at meals perfectly naturally and frankly and decently about the work. Of course if a lay person were inside for five minutes they'd be horrified. But it's just because they go on like this that horrid jokes or anything approaching to sex doesn't come into the question at all.

It's most dear of you to send the cheque.

Your very loving O.W.

July 25

Belovedest Monna,

This only a line, because at a case since 6.30 this morning (breakfastless, lunchless till half hour ago). Most interesting case but, as usual, abnormal to the last degree! After getting help and the woman having forceps, haemorrhage and God knows what other complications, I now have to say that she and the boy are both alive – the latter lustily, the former as near dead as she can be. I've now had seven cases and devil a one of normal use to me. Isn't it sickening? I'm so tired of these strangenesses.

Can't now dine with Lady Arnott tonight – must go and see this nice woman late this evening as she had a devilish time. We agreed it must be a boy, because he was so tedious keeping her hanging about so long. It's a fact, you know, that boys give more trouble, God knows why – except the general lack of consideration which is always greater in any boy than a girl. Tiresome little brutes. Her name is Bridget Lyons, bright red hair, thirty-three, seventh pregnancy. It's the devil to see the pain these women suffer. An old towel is tied to the top of the bed which they can pull at, and the sweat pours off them – their hair gets drenched, they groan and gasp, they put the towel between their teeth and bite it as they pull, for very agony. All this perhaps for ten hours, some much less, others more. And it's just the devil. The more you bear down and strain the faster you get a move on the baby but the more hellish pain you get. And they almost all work like niggers. But it's heartbreaking to watch, and they so grateful for the nothing you do. Last night (other case) the baby was going to be called Patrick Pearce after the Sinn Fein martyr!

I've just about had enough of watching pain and suffering, so it's getting quite hard to believe in anything good – without your letters I'd run away!

Your very own   O.W.

Never a 'child' any more is this one. One's only a child as long as one's more or less ignorant of some of the misery and filth of this world. Thank heaven you never did go in for Medicine. I couldn't bear for you to be doing some of these things.

Saturday 7.30a.m.

All the infants I bring into the world are going to be called Michael – except the ones called after Sinn Fein martyrs! Likewise, you'll observe, they're all boys which makes the mothers often pleased with me and call me 'lucky' to them, which is thoroughly against all my principles, as they ought to be just as ready to have girls. What fairly shocks me is the way women of twenty-seven look about fifty here – I suppose it's all the childbearing which does it. Never have I seen so many children in the streets in any town. No birth control here because it's against the Roman Catholic religion.

Eighth baby. Yesterday morning I was hailed out.

July 30

I got one and a half hours of sleep this morning. At breakfast Dr English: 'Would you like to help at operations this morning?'

'Oh yes, very much,' says O.W. As a rule only qualified people allowed to. I don't know whether this was arranged on purpose or not, in the hope that I'd be paid out. Jellett has the devil's temper, this morning; the real theatre sister away for holiday and the biggest fool taking her place. The operation in question one of the biggest in gynaecology. O.W.'s preparation a night of stress and little sleep. I was upstairs preparing to wash up. Comes along Jellett: 'What are you here for?'

O.W. 'I've the honour of assisting you operate this morning.' Mebbe he thought it cheek, but I actually meant what I said.

'Well, but have you ever helped before at *big* operations?'

O.W. 'Oh yes, not here, but in London.'

'But it's very tiring; your back will be broken; it may take quite three hours!'

O.W. 'Oh my back won't break, sir,' and I laughed.

Now, everybody operates differently, uses different tools, likes different ways. However, says I to myself, this is obviously Jellett's first experience of women and he's mightily unwilling and distrustful of them. Also, those beastly men have probably arranged this just so I should make a fool of myself and get sworn at. He asked me the names of one or two arteries and I made vile mistakes. However, we operated for two-and-a-half hours solid and I can't say I wasn't thankful when it was over because the effort of it was mighty strenuous. But he didn't swear at me and twice he said he was either being very silly or very stupid in not achieving something in two minutes which he took nearly forty-five over (as a matter of fact anybody would, it was a nasty job). But I think I wasn't too clumsy and I thought that remark looked as if he thought I was grown up enough to understand and perchance criticise his work. Of course I'm not. I believe I'm getting some hang of this show.

Your very loving S.C.

July 30

Darling, things may be interesting here. Some of my patients are Sinn Feiners, others have brothers and sisters who are. They tell me on all sides that on Sunday and possibly on August bank holiday there's likely to be trouble. It is supposed that the military will fire on them and clear them out neck and crop – for my part I think they'll be arrested in groups and drastic measures will be necessary. Now, my information comes solely from the poor, from my patients who, one and all I think I can truthfully say, are attached to me; hence they tell me almost any blessed thing – a great deal more, in fact, than I can digest, they're so eloquent! If by chance there should be bloodshed and fighting again, this hospital is not likely to suffer because it entirely shelters the poor. They don't as a rule violate hospitals, and everybody of the poor I've met so far has a most exalted view of the medical profession (unlike the average English and American!). I have no fear at all of any violence so long as I have my little professional bag in the streets of Dublin. So if aught happens please don't be agitated. At the Arnotts the other day they'd been having all the generals in command to dine and there are enough troops and ammunition in Ireland to settle the biggest rising; since, however, the Sinn Feiners have no ammunition now there simply can't be much fight.

Tonight Bellows has a case. Been on all day. I examined her and the whole hospital are agog about her because it's a face presentation. I'd never felt one before but I was sure it was – everybody would like to be there, as they are rare but you go only by invite to another's case, so of course I'll have first look in with Bellows. Indeed, she asked me if she got fussed about the case and anxious might she send for me?! Dunderdale today said it had been an education last night to see how I dealt with the patient, how calm and unfussing I was, calculated to inspire confidence generally!

July 31

Face case not come off yet and infant now died, I'm afraid, in utero. We still await the birth which is bound to be interesting. Today I went off and watched Sir Arthur Ball operate this morning. Awfully nice little man, treated me like a colleague, explained the case to me, showed me round afterwards. He says there are often rumours of Sinn Fein trouble but they don't come to anything, so this will probably be like the rest.

Been 'fitten and quorlin' with Bellows. I'm so very glad I'm at a mixed hospital. Controversy was this: The face case baby having died, Bellows told Simpson (Assistant Master) about it. 'Serves her right, she should have come into hospital. After one takes all the trouble to get a woman pregnant, the least she can do is to come into hospital for her confinement.' She had been told to do so, because she had to have treatment in the first place to make childbearing possible and therefore she needed watching. But they're beastly obstinate, these people and think they'll be as well looked after in their own homes. Now Simpson made that remark because he was furious at the baby dying. He minds terribly when they do. But he's Irish and says things like that without altogether meaning them literally.

Bellows fired up furiously, 'Oh you are a brute, *I wish you men could have babies for a year or two.*' He became quite scarlet, said nothing, tho' he was plainly near to murdering her. So, says I after to her that she didn't ought *ever* to make a remark like the underlined part. It's not the thing. If you go in for Medicine you've simply got to forget the differences in sex, else you'll make the whole work impossible. I can't tell you how damaging to women's doing Medicine is a remark as personal as that – it affects the whole foundation of things and is the worst possible taste. Of course it nearly makes me personally feel I don't want to associate with anybody who has that type of mind, because it harms the status of medical women so much – it's the Almroth Wright touch. So I just mentioned gently that I thought it a mistake (as she has made that same remark before) and she is simply furious with me. But I don't think she'll do it again, which is a net gain.

By the end of yesterday's operation Jellett had forgotten

he'd got a girl helping him – and that's what I'd always hope
any male colleague would feel if I were working with him.
And it was quite a step for Jellett in the educational line, so
I do want to achieve the same with his Assistant Masters here
too. It all helps to consolidate women's position in Medicine.
Dr English, the Clinical Clerk, is being quite civil and
instructive and beginning to feel that one may have some
brains for the job. That too is a step. He took about ten
minutes examining the face case (I'd taken about two) and
I'd told him before I took him out to see the case what I
thought. But he didn't listen much since all students feel the
queerest inaccurate things. However, he turned round and
asked me did I think the chin was anterior and it came to me
that my diagnosis had a little surprised him by its accuracy.
So we've got to consolidate our position as *medical*
colleagues, and not go sliding back into 'girls' and personalities. I personally think it easy to achieve the former,
so I hate when people go and put the clock back.

Midnight Saturday

About the Bellows-Simpson incident. I obviously didn't
retail it accurately for you. Simpson is an odd man – very
capable and good at his job. He hates hurting people. I was
watching him today at a protracted labour and that man
simply suffered. When he made that remark the other day
about Bellows's case he was furious because he thought the
child's life had been sacrificed, and the woman had brought
upon herself unnecessary pain and suffering by not coming
into hospital. The other day I discovered he'd spent fifty
minutes persuading a woman to have hospital treatment in
order that her life might be prolonged. You don't find
London doctors 'wasting' time that way.

None of these men here have ever made any remark such
as I seem to have wrongly conveyed the impression to you.
They're awfully kind and considerate to the patients in their
different ways, and they're looked up to all over Dublin
wherever I go. And nothing has ever been said in bad taste

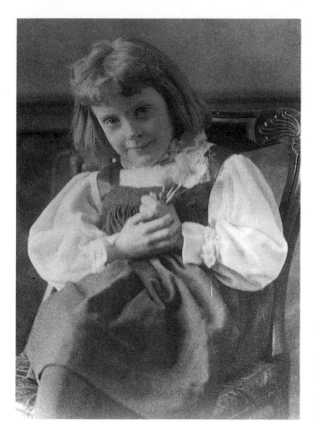

(left) Octavia Wilberforce as a child.

(below) Octavia's mother, Mrs Anna Wilberforce.

(below left) Octavia's father, Reginald Garton Wilberforce.

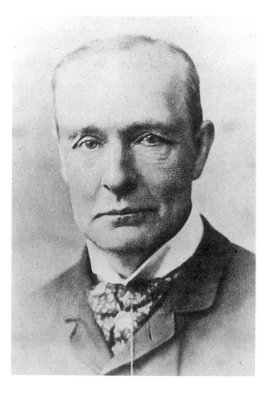

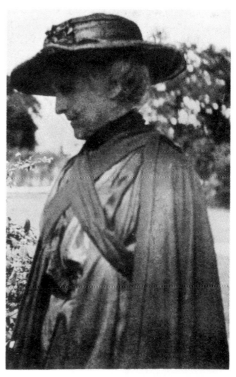

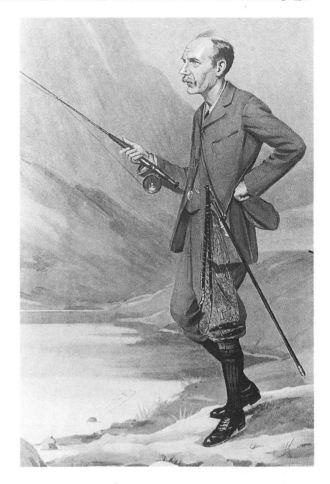

(above) An old map of
Lavington Manor, from the
family house.

(right) Sydney (later Lord)
Buxton, Postmaster-General in
the Liberal Government
of 1912–13.

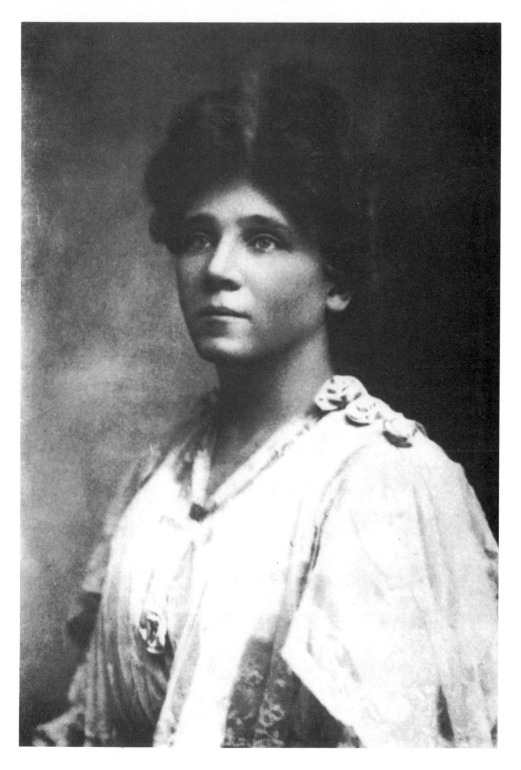

Elizabeth Robins

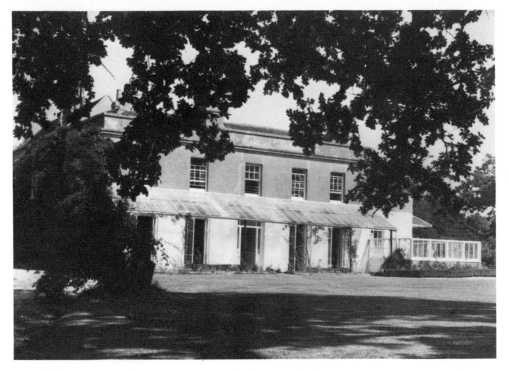

(above) Bramlands, near Henfield in Sussex, was
Elizabeth Robins' home in 1909.

(below) Backsettown, the fifteenth-century Sussex
farmhouse where Elizabeth Robins lived and which she
and Octavia Wilberforce turned into a convalescent
home for women after 1927.

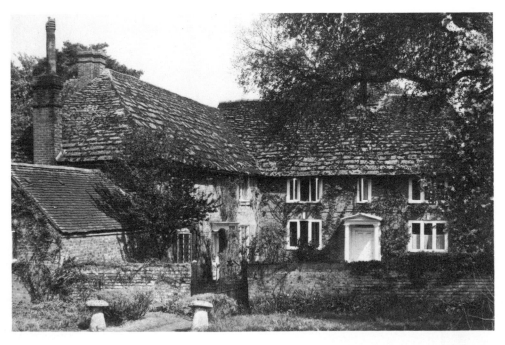

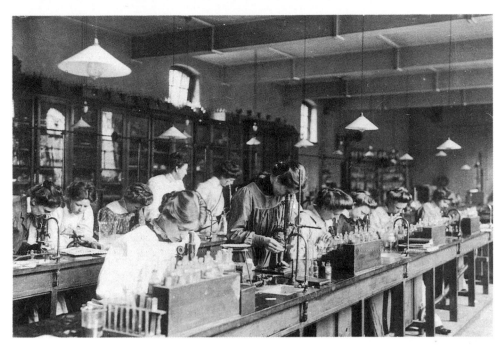

(above) Students at work in the laboratory at the London School of Medicine for Women, which Octavia attended from 1913–20.

(below) Midwifery students at the Rotunda Hospital in Dublin, where Octavia worked as a junior doctor from 1920-22.

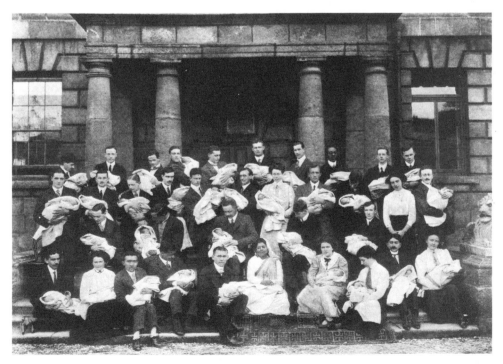

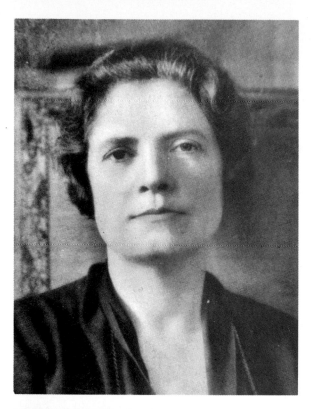

(*left*) Margaret Haig, Viscountess Rhondda. She was the editor of the radical journal *Time and Tide*, which campaigned vigorously for women's suffrage – and herself successfully fought for the right to take her seat in the House of Lords.

(*below left*) The statue of William Wilberforce in Westminster Abbey and (*below right*) Octavia Wilberforce dressed in her great-grandfather's Court dress.

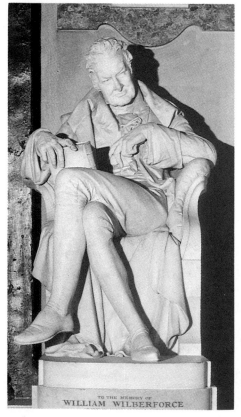

TO THE MEMORY OF
WILLIAM WILBERFORCE

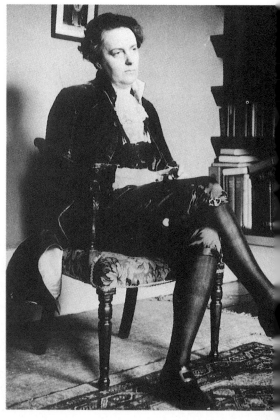

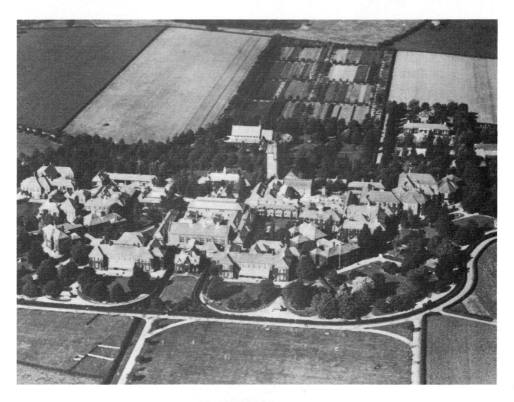

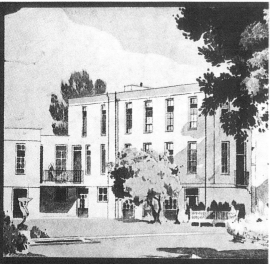

The New Sussex Hospital
for Women and Children
BRIGHTON
(Incorporated)

(above) Graylingwell Hospital, in West Sussex. While working with mental patients there, Octavia became struck by the number of professional single women under care.

(left) Brochure for the New Sussex Hospital for Women and Children, where Octavia worked from 1923 until her retirement.

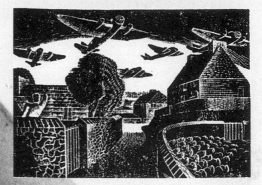

(above) Virginia Woolf.

(right) Report of Virginia Woolf's disappearance from the Brighton *Evening Argus*, 3 April 1941.

(inset above) Contemporary woodcut of the Woolfs' home, Monks House, Rodmell, Sussex, during a German raid. According to Octavia Wilberforce, it was the anxiety of wartime that triggered Virginia Woolf's final suicidal depression.

MISSING AUTHORESS

Sussex River Dragged

UNAVAILING search has been made of the countryside around Rodmell for Mrs. Virginia Woolf, the authoress, who disappeared from her Rodmell home on Friday last, and the River Ouse in the vicinity has been dragged, without result.

The river is tidal at the point where Mrs. Woolf is believed to have disappeared.

Mrs. Woolf was very fond of walking alongside the Ouse.

Her husband told a reporter last night: "Mrs. Woolf is presumed to be dead. She went for a walk on Friday leaving a letter behind and it is thought she has been drowned. Her body has, however, not been recovered."

Daughter of the late Sir Leslie Stephen, K.C.B., a distinguished man of letters, Mrs. Virginia Woolf married Mr. Leonard Sidney Woolf, Joint Editor of the Political Quarterly, and in 1917 they collaborated in founding the Hogarth Press, a publishing firm from the partnership of which Mrs. Woolf retired in 1938 to devote her time to writing.

It is said that Mr. and Mrs. Woolf began the firm with a second-hand printing press bought in a rag and bone shop.

Mrs. Woolf, with her sister, the artist Vanessa, founded the old Bloomsbury Group. Her later books, which attracted considerable attention, were "The Years," "Three Guineas," "Reviewing" and a biography of Roger Fry.

about any case here. And I seem thoroughly to have given you a wrong impression, so please take it off.

The best part of this place is the way men and women work together, and the younger men, Simpson, Gilmour, English, feel one just as capable as the men students. It's only Jellett who thinks one may be frailer, but he's the older generation. Jellett plays up to and half flirts with every girl. Bellows, who is essentially a flirt, adores him and plays to catch his eye. These younger men don't want to flirt but do want to help one all they can. Here in Dublin, men and women students have worked together at Trinity College for years. At Arthur Ball's hospital I was so pleased to see the perfect naturalness and equality of men and women. They forget half the time that there's any difference between the men and women students, and that's what you need in Medicine. Equality and absence of sex.

I'd willingly tell any man he was a beast if I thought he was being heartless or indecent about a woman, but I'd *never* introduce as an argument that he *being a man* couldn't understand anything about having babies. I've never had babies either, but it doesn't mean that I, any more than Simpson, am ignorant of the pain it involves. And I'd certainly never own that I was incapable of understanding about or ministering to some of the ailments peculiar to men. No man doctor has ever hinted at such a possibility; they take it for granted one suffers in imagination easily enough the various pains one's patients undergo. Suppose you said I couldn't conceive what Janet suffered because I hadn't tuberculosis, I'd feel exceedingly angry. Understanding of pain in Medicine is not limited to experience or sex – else nobody would ever progress. And even to bring differences of sex or physical disabilities of women into any argument, is playing the Almroth Wright, Freudian, sex mad note and I simply detest it.

I'm all in favour of women treating women if they prefer it, and men treating men if they prefer it. But I'll never own that I'd be incapable of treating men's diseases with every bit as good results as the men get. A doctor is one whose primary use is to heal. The age, religion, political opinions, sex, colour of skin of his patient are all immaterial and I entirely refuse to have limits imposed in any direction!

Ye Gods, it *is* interesting here, there's no doubt as to that. By the way, Bellows said afterwards to me she greatly regretted losing her temper. Simpson, however, bore no ill-will – people don't and he realised she'd had no sleep. She didn't realise that he had been cursing in the porter's lodge at midnight the previous night at not having been sent for to deal with that very same woman!

Bless you my darling.

Your birthday. 3 p.m.

[Octavia argued in this letter that the advantages of her acting as Elizabeth Robins's literary agent outweighed the disadvantages:]

There are two things to be said, I feel.

1. Which is against:

It is always rather a question, I think, whether having money and business dealings with somebody doesn't poison a personal relationship – I do wonder about that? Suppose, too, I went and did something foolish? (tho' personally I don't feel anything but confident about being able to do the job efficiently and successfully once I'd got two or three things clear). You'd be terribly and justifiably annoyed but I so much dislike any reproof from you and feel it so acutely that I'd never dare be a fool I'm thinking!

2. If you gave me half the commission you give Watt it might keep me out of the workhouse. Suppose Phyllis pays no more fees for me? [after her forthcoming marriage to Ponsonby]. I wrote long ago about them and have heard never a word. It's more than likely he's not a sixpence and anyhow people in love are utterly unreliable in such matters. Therefore I'd simply love to *earn* some money and I really feel I conscientiously would be able to do the business for you once I picked up the ropes. I'm quick at practical things like that.

I believe I could do it well and save you money. Could save you trouble and would be really grateful for the chance of earning some money. My 'time'. Please, beloved, don't think about that. I'd simply love to do it and it wouldn't interfere with my medical works at all. Why Humphry Ward doesn't do anything but his wife's agenting; by the way, later on why not have him to tea or something and let him explain to me?! Is that a preposterous idea? I'm really quite good at dealing with business things, and it would be a great experience and adventure to do. By all means I'll deal with advertisements, but not a penny's commission will I receive, indeed no. Wouldn't do it on that understanding at all. It's a purely personal thing which gives me pleasure to do as it saves you trouble. Also not the same bother and effort for me as for you.

Your very, very own most loving,
Sussex Child

August 7 1918

I wonder whether you've gathered that I'm immensely happy in my work here and simply love it in so far as being of real use is concerned. I'm not loving midwifery especially (not that branch of Medicine), but the dealing with patients and getting 'em better, and the responsibility and the way it stirs one up to think of things to help. I revel in all that.

I was fearfully pleased today. A woman said a neighbour in some house was expecting baby next week. Might they send specially for me rather than any other doctor? Now you'll go and think that's because I'm good at the job. I tell you probably I'm not, but I'm generally fairly good in giving the mother confidence and reassuring her. That's why they like me, Monna beloved, and the value of it is not much, tho' a little.

Only the one baby died (seven months one, and they always do unless incubated or nearly roasted by a fire). Else the rest of my patients are (I touch wood) most well and healthy. I fight them all as regards when they get up. They all want to get up very soon and I adopt various devices for making them have just a little longer in bed – different temperaments want different treatment mentally. (Bellows interrupts to say doesn't this work make me want to have a baby. When I say, 'No, it does *not*.' she opens wide eyes and fails by leagues to understand. We'll talk about this one day, you and I, just so you won't misunderstand my views.) With some, one tells them they mustn't get up for eleven days or so, knowing that they'll then sneak out about the eighth – so one allows for it. With others one keeps them in bed by constant visiting and more or less intimidation! It's very interesting all this side of the matter.

[This morning the mother] needed stitching. When I told her this (they often refuse), she said 'Will you do it yourself, doctor?' and I said 'Yes', she again impressed on me that I personally had to do the job. I was quite flattered. Tonight when I get round to her again and did the stitch, she said I hardly hurt at all. It's the most damnably painful job imaginable, so I think it was really nice of her.

Each day is one rush. Lucky if the nights aren't too. So it's just no good trying to fit in outside things as well. Tomorrow I may go to tea with Balls again and thence to see over Trinity College with Sir Arthur. He's a dear and asked me to see him operate this morning, but I only got back at quarter to ten, and class on at ten, and I'm tired (in legs), so I hadn't the energy; else I love watching other people operate and seeing other hospitals.

Your Sussex Child

August 10 8 a.m. At a case

Another primapara. Far the most interesting and difficult. Yesterday, went to one at 3.30, girl of twenty-six, thoroughly obstreperous and tiresome – would keep clutching my arm when I was all washed up. Had to be rather severe with her, and tell her she would poison herself. Of course it paid. I hate doing it when they're having pains and suffering, but it's the only thing, for their good, to be firm and, if necessary, cross. Result always the same with these Irish. They are the biggest babies ever born (the mothers) and are quite good and like one immensely if one is stern with them.

The one yesterday tried to interfere while the baby was being born, so I had to speak severely to her. Afterwards the placenta wouldn't come away. One is supposed to send in to hospital after three quarters of an hour if it doesn't arrive. I waited one and a quarter hours doing all I could. Nothing happened. So I sent in a form and the angelic Dr English came out in a car to the rescue – nice of him not to waste time as it was a long way off and he kept the car too (which was better still) to go back in. He got the thing away successfully (and we got back at nine). He was duly pleased at the fact that, tho' she was a primapara, I hadn't let the perineum tear. This last is far more likely to happen in the primapara, so I too was very pleased. Many of the multiparae lately have torn because I wasn't good at it and because they'd all been torn before – so this was really better.

Dashed back to breakfast. Hardly swallowed it when sent for again. Case came off at 12. A good case, only blowed if placenta didn't get stuck again. It was still immovable after two hours, so again English was involved. He laughed, but was quite nice about it and thoroughly impressed at the perineum again being untorn, the more so since he saw the size of the boy's head. Not only impressed but surprised at the fact. Blinked: 'That's good. I say, you're rather an expert over these,' and on the way back asked how many cases I'd had externally – evidently wondering how I'd managed to get so good at it. O.W. thoroughly pleased. Two labours, two days running, both primaparae and both 'perineum intact' – to enter in the annals of the hospital. Getting rather set up, ma'am.

I wish I could hear from Phyllis. I certainly ought to have by now, but I suppose an event like marriage entirely puts out of mind every ordinary friend one has. All the more vital therefore that I did some agenting for you. Thrilling about Thring not altogether disapproving of my agenting. I'd love to do it. And these agents do seem to be robbers, don't they?

Saturday

There's no doubt as to my need of sleep, nor my appreciation of flealess nights. Till I'd been to Dublin I'd never been grateful enough for unbitten nights.

By the way, I have to eat my words re the disgustingness of this special branch of Medicine. I thought it a horrid, messy job and hated it at first, but really it's the most attractive and gratifying of any branch of healing. For this reason. You have a patient more or less ailing for nine months, at the end of her pregnancy definitely ill, and having about the worst pain that's known. (Every woman varies, but most educated ones will tell you – if they see you before they mercifully forget the anguish of it – that having teeth out without gas is like child's play in comparison.) These pains may go on for thirty hours intermittently at the end. You do your job. And after an hour they say they feel 'grand' and they do in comparison to the days before.

Now, there's no other piece of Medicine or Surgery where you get such quick results for your trouble and that's why Martindale and such-like love the work. They make well in record time, and God knows, to anybody who goes in for healing, the patience and endless time it generally takes to cure people; this is a vast contrast. And therefore, my darling, I personally feel that a little midwifery thrown into my work would be most gratifying and consoling. Indeed I would like having a piece of a hospital devoted to it under my care. Only I've no wish to attend the people in their own homes specially (not the poor). It seems to me the risk of sepsis is too great (tho' none of my Dublin patients were so afflicted, I must admit). But still, if you have fleas and lice hopping over everything, you ought to get septic unless you're lucky – so it's a risk that is needless. Also, incidentally, it's a nice work as regards your use mentally to the patients. I mean if you've any gift for inspiring confidence you'll help the patient vastly over this 'illness'.

Your very own most loving,

S.C.

On the return journey the Irish Channel was very rough. My travelling co-student left me lying down below, dismally seasick. Earlier in the year, when lunching at Lady Brassey's, she told of a relative in the Mediterranean who, though a bad sailor, was completely stopped from being seasick when the ship was fired on by Germans. Fear had ousted the seasickness. I was being disgustingly afflicted and felt perfectly awful when I became aware of sudden intense activity and footsteps overhead. Bellows, my Rotunda co-student, dashed in.

'Put on your lifebelt – the periscope of a German submarine is sighted on the horizon and we'll probably be torpedoed.'

I groaned, 'I don't care. I can't move. Go away.' She became very angry but couldn't get any sense into my head. Finally she left me feeling I would welcome any torpedo. I remember it took me two days to recover when I arrived back in London and Mrs Ware, the landlady at Cambridge Terrace, was much concerned! So much for cure by Fear.

8

DIVIDED INTERESTS

Surgery Versus Lady Rhondda and Time and Tide

1918–20

I spent the next two years in the wards. More and more men students came back to their changed hospital, where they found women not only as students but actually as residents in several of the house posts. The majority bore it with equanimity because they had come to know something of the good work done by women in the war. The hospital authorities had at first said that the women couldn't possibly share the residents' quarters with the men. It was unheard of in those days that they should use the same bathrooms and WCs. The difficulties were finally overcome by one bathroom being reserved for women exclusively, and the situation came to be generally accepted.

The summer holiday of 1918 was unforgettable. It was Lady Rhondda who suggested we should go to Wales and see Snowdon. Beddgelert was decided upon. After a few days of trying to climb with skirts, I suggested we should do better in Land Army breeches, to which E.R. agreed, and I wrote for outfits on approval. We would leave the hotel looking quite ladylike in the long skirts of those days. After half a mile or so we would discard the skirts, put them into my rucksack, and continue with ecstatic freedom in the Land Army breeches which were concealed underneath. One day we took the little train up Snowdon, and ate our sandwiches on the summit, enjoying its magnificent views. Then we began our two-hour walk down the Rhyd-ddu path in perfect weather, and arrived at Pits Head to wait for a bus, but this was long in coming and E.R. was tired out. I caught sight of a traction engine lumbering and puffing towards us, and accosted the kindly Welsh driver who allowed us to ride home with the boxes of ginger beer and such like. A great day, and beyond being burnt to the hue of lobsters, we were not a penny the worse.

I was due to take my examination for Medicine in January 1919 when I developed appalling earache. My terror of the examination was nearly wiped out by an equal fear that I might be unable to take it. A furuncle complicated by wax was diagnosed and in spite of treatment the pain continued. I managed to sit but felt very ill, and was afraid I had failed. The viva was still before me. The pain had eliminated all fear and made me completely reckless. One of the questions asked for in writing was treatment for hypertension. I dashed off quite a long answer, and ended by saying that I would send the patient to Woodhall Spa. The elderly, distinguished consultant who examined me in the viva looked at me sarcastically: 'And why Woodhall Spa, may I ask? Have you shares in it?' My ear was giving me spasms of pain, I felt this was an insulting question, and I lost my temper and became completely fluent. 'The water has iodides in it,' I said indignantly, and added a whole lot about the benefit of spas, and getting away from home responsibilities. He had to cut me short and proceeded to ask me other questions. Savagely and furiously I answered them, having unwontedly no difficulty in either producing or marshalling the necessary facts. I returned to Cambridge Street still angry, and had more drops and treatment for several days. It was finally discovered I had a perforation, and I was ordered three weeks off duty. Then the results came through – I had passed! The first time, too, which was astounding. Looking back I attribute this success not only to my insatiable interest in pure Medicine, but to the earache which caused my examination apprehensions to be eliminated by rage!

E.R. and Dr Martindale, a forceful combination, sent me to a nursing home in Brighton for which E.R. paid. I was tended by Dr Martindale, rested and fed up. 'Fed up' in more than one sense as I was soon tired of bed, and became yet more tired of nursing home treatment and food. I went to Backset for a couple of days to revel in freedom after the nursing home routine, and then back to London to prepare for the examination in Pharmacy, which I also passed successfully. Surgery was still before me, but the Surgery demonstrations I often found dull, because I knew I did not want to become a surgeon. I determined to concentrate on Medicine, for Dr Sydney Phillips's time at St Mary's Hospital was coming to an end and I was determined to cherish every smallest clinical crumb that fell from his lips. My absorption of Surgery naturally suffered. Dr Phillips lectured on the infectious nature of the fell disease, originally termed Spanish influenza; he told how two young men who had recovered from the complaint returned after convalescence to their lodgings to the same pillows and blankets, and went down with it again the night of their return. It taught me always to stress the importance of fresh bedding if possible. He was a man after my own heart, with a twinkle in his deep-set dark eyes. He would say, 'I always tease my surgical colleagues and tell them all that is needed to be a first-class surgeon is to be a good French dressmaker. They never like it.'

E.R. was busy over plans for the New Sussex Hospital. She was at that time chairman and called upon Sir Hugh Bell and other friends to subscribe. The site behind the old Windlesham House in Brighton, which had been a boys' school, was considered ideal for the hospital, and Mrs Yates Thompson anonymously gave the money to buy it. This was a great step forward. Lady Rhondda consented to become the first honorary treasurer, and at a meeting at the Rendels in the spring of 1919 she gave £500. Mr Clayton, the architect, was hard at work on ambitious plans.

Lady Rhondda was a romantic figure, for she had been torpedoed in the *Lusitania* and such a miraculous escape seemed to mark her out for a special destiny. She was full of ideas about the position and potential power of women in the world. E.R. immediately responded to her approach and we saw a great deal of her, both in London and at Backset, where she came to stay. When, as often happened, E.R. was not available, Lady Rhondda would take me off for walks and endless discussions. I liked her immensely, and much sympathised with her fervour to write and her battle to be allowed to take her seat in the House of Lords; and [also] with the idea that she might produce an independent, unbiased periodical [*Time and Tide*] which would be directed by a picked body of distinguished women who would give confidence to women readers. How best could all this be achieved, and would E.R. help to interest her friends and introduce Lady Rhondda to future contributors? Endless talks followed and many plans were laid. Lady Rhondda expressed herself earnestly and fluently, and her steady, enquiring gaze, her sudden smile and rather low voice, with its slight difficulty over the R's, made her peculiarly attractive.

At that time hospital work was making ever greater demands and I was rather torn by divided interests. Lady Rhondda was going through a bad patch and reported to E.R. that *Time and Tide* had cost her £6800 in one month. Then, coming out with Lady Bell, after seeing Sybil Thorndike in *The Trojan Women*, E.R. was confronted by newspapermen with a placard in huge letters, 'Lady Rhondda's Wrecked Happiness'. The paper was full of the pending divorce.

On 4 May 1919, E.R. gave a dinner party at her club to the Buxtons, Lady Rhondda and her mother, Lord Ernle, Herbert Richmond, Mark Milbanke, and Lord Robert Cecil. The next morning E.R. was visited at her club while still in bed (an almost unpardonable interruption) by Lady Rhondda, who was going to the United States of America and wanted advice as to where to go for a retreat. Then she asked, possibly the real cause of her visit, if E.R. thought she ought to go to the House of Lords tomorrow, as the petition for her to inherit her father's seat was then to be considered. She claimed that peeresses should have this right. On this she was met by a very firm 'Certainly' from E.R. They had quite an argument about it and finally she accepted the advice, but what should she wear? She gravely discussed three possible gowns. E.R. plumped for the 'newest, smartest and best' and was engaged to go and support her. Next day at 10.15 E.R. was met at the House of Lords by Lady Rhondda and her mother and was taken to Black Rod's box. On the way they met Lord Buxton who was rather embarrassed for he was no advocate of women's emancipation. She was introduced to Lady Rhondda's KC, Talbot, and her solicitor. There then ensued a duel between the Lord Chancellor, F.E. Smith, and Talbot, with interruptions from Lords Haldane, Carson, Phillimore, Finlay, and Buckmaster, amongst others. After lunch they returned to the House of Lords, and F.E. Smith, after a good lunch, was still more annoyed and spiky. There was an adjournment at quarter to four and Talbot thought they would throw out Lady Rhondda's petition, [as they did]. With the failure of the petition, E.R. wrote articles for the papers on the House of Lords, but Lady Rhondda was convinced that the press was against her. E.R. did all she could to help her and Lady Rhondda appreciated it.

Lady Rhondda wrote to E.R. in August 1919:

> I have been thinking of that problem of the co-ordination of woman-power all these last few months and I have a scheme in my head which I think might help – the gist of it all is the need for the Trade Union spirit.

When Lady Rhondda returned from the United States of America she was full of new ideas. I am amused to find that, with the arrogance and assurance of the reasonably young, I did my best to teach her about some aspects of modern medicine over which she held old-fashioned views. I also argued with her about Freud and did my best to enlighten her on the subject of the menopause. It is entertaining to see the violence of the impact of Freud's doctrines on two young women at that period.

Grand Hotel des Alpes
Murren

2.1.20.

You'll be glad to hear that your letter has had a certain effect on my mistaken views [on the menopause]. I still think that you are veering too much the other way, but after all, if your job in life is going to be to do away with the old prejudices about it, I suppose you are almost bound to exaggerate on the other side. Still I do find it impossible to believe that such a big change as comes to women doesn't show at all in their general health, balance and nerves – especially when one knows that one's period does affect one quite considerably sometimes.

I'll admit it's probably grossly exaggerated at present and you medical women have a lot to do yet in that direction – but I can't believe it's non-existent – that doesn't seem to me possible. I wouldn't like to dismiss it as non-existent unless it really were, because it's surely sounder to face facts. However, perhaps you'll convince me yet, you've certainly shaken me a bit!

Rhondda

20.7.20

Dear Miss Wilberforce,

Do you think that if all goes well in the autumn I could ask Miss Robins whether she would let us have the serial rights of her next book [for *Time and Tide*]? We would pay whatever other people do of course (if we could afford to ask her at all) but I am not sure whether it would be awful cheek asking her for a little, unknown paper like ours. Only we do feel that – as she says herself – we ought to get all the outstanding women to write in our paper, and make it really a selection of the very best of what women are doing.

Yours, Rhondda

17.8.20

My dear Octavia,

I don't think you were in the least rude! Anyhow not nearly as rude as I was! The fact was we were shocking the other horribly! I you by having read Freud. You me by seeming to uphold the theory which I hate most in the world: 'This must be left to those who know.' I needn't explain how entirely I disagree with the theory that sex or psychology lie any more within the medical man's province than they do within any one else's. You speak as if only a doctor knew the laws and punishments nature has created 'in self defence against sex'. But after all it's the business of all educated people to know them. And certainly those of us who went through the Suffrage Movement learnt of those punishments in every circumstantial and unpleasant detail.

But to try and suppress Freud because you detest him – that is indeed 'allowing hugely for sex'; it's admitting you're afraid of it. Why you're as bad as the old people who wouldn't admit religious doubt. We'll never make a clean world by being afraid to tackle anything in heaven or earth. And you'll never get sex into its right proportion if you put a veil round it and say 'Please don't look.' As a matter of fact, these folk like Freud (or Forel or Havelock Ellis) are just the people who are likely to have the result of reducing sex to smaller proportions. It's the 'pretty pretty' treatment that keeps it big.

Yours, M.

24.8.20
My dear Octavia,

Just a line to say I'm feeling rather ashamed of myself for being so cantankerous. What I ought to have told you at the time was that I never did believe in Freud's sex theories. What one admires about the man and what interests one is that he is trying to push back the frontiers of knowledge in rather a new way and in (to some extent) a new direction. He seems to have brought new system to an old unsystematised branch of knowledge and I feel he will be remembered for that. It's the men who come after him who will make the real discoveries. I don't think books do affect me enormously – or at least not Freud's sex. I'd thought and read too much about it before to take a new impression very easily.

Yours, M.

I've a feeling that these outside social activities, combined with constant concern with domestic staff, must have contributed quite a lot to my inability to absorb Surgery for examination purposes. We had moved from 6 Cambridge Terrace, as some Australian friends of Mrs Ward's had made a tempting offer for eighteen months for our rooms. Our new lodging at No. 78 gave no 'attendance', and we had to rely on 'chars', as they were then designated. They didn't turn up, they objected to E.R.'s high standard of cleanliness, or their little boys developed mumps, so that quite often we, and particularly I, had to turn to and cook and char. On occasions the good-hearted Mrs Ward would come in and rescue the situation if we were expecting a visitor to dinner – Rose Macaulay or William Archer, perhaps, who wanted to discuss literary matters peacefully with E.R.

I had not been very fit during the winter of 1919 and early 1920 and I had failed in Surgery. It was then that Lady Bell invited me to Rounton for a holiday. As a piece of what would now be termed Occupational Therapy, E.R. and I thought of writing together a cookery book for children to be used as a serial for *Time and Tide*, which by now had started publication. It proved an interesting distraction, and I used to cook each dish at Backset before we incorporated the recipe into the story. I had, too, devoted a little of my time to writing a semi-medical article: 'More rest better work' for *Time and Tide*. It was of course unsigned. I also wrote one on the eighteen-year-old Joyce Wetherhed, who had snatched the golf championship from the holder, Miss Leitch. These articles and my share in *Prudence and Peter* were the only earned money I had so far received. It was distinctly stimulating.

The flat at 78 Cambridge Terrace had been sublet, so Lady Rhondda generously lent me her quiet and spacious flat at 15 Chelsea Court, overlooking the Embankment, for the last weeks before my next Surgery examination in September 1920. There was the unprecedented luxury of a first-rate, kind maid to come in and 'do' for me. Never had I studied with such a minimum of distraction.

I had twice failed the Surgery examination and found it hard to memorise facts in Surgical anatomy. Mr (subsequently Sir) Zachary Cope was the only surgeon whose lectures I found easy to pay attention to. Once again I had recourse to private coaching, first from Professor Ida Mann (later Ophthalmic Consultant to the Government of Western Australia) who had a brain capable of memorising three or four pages of *Gray's Anatomy* at one reading. Later Mr Gordon Bryan, a thickset, perhaps slower-geared, patient individual who laboured earnestly to hammer in surgical anatomy facts and operative surgery descriptions. He explained that the examiners had raised the standard, especially for women, 'because they are not so precise'. It is my belief now that he rather cleverly went out of his way to say things to rouse me so that I had to accustom myself to answer back, which is what examiners like. He told me that men were governed by their intellect whereas women were governed by their emotions. This stung me to ask: 'Then you don't think women will ever make good doctors?'

'No,' he replied, 'they haven't the physique.' Fortunately, his job was to teach me Surgery; mine wasn't to educate him to more enlightened views! I liked him for his absolutely impersonal method in teaching one all about the many sexual things one had to know. Some people left them out, others did it heroically, and hated the effort, or, worse still, enjoyed doing it, which made one uncomfortable.

The weeks at Chelsea Court were rewarding. I passed Surgery and was at last qualified to embark on the sea of Medicine. What a final triumph, and how elated was E.R. Even Mr Bryan was pleased and seemed to think my future was assured. Pam was delighted, and asked me to dine in celebration. Lord Buxton congratulated me and most generously said he would continue my allowance (£100 a year) for the first six months after qualification. [He wrote:] 'It has been a real pleasure and now also a satisfaction – for your sake and Phyllis's – to have been able to help you at all.'

[At this turning point in her life, Octavia paused to assess the importance and the nature of her relationship with Elizabeth Robins:]

I was immeasurably blessed in having E.R.'s steadfast affection and unquenchable faith in my ultimate success. Her association with me over those long struggling years was essentially a maternal one – protective, far-seeing, ambitious for my success. 'Essentially maternal' may seem an odd term to apply to a very close friendship, but E.R. was possessed of acutely sensitive antennae. [She had] gained an insight into the maintenance of a close, abiding, loving tie which was never possessive in hampering my professional career. That she worried about my constant colds and throats did not make her want to exert pressure when I firmly wished to pursue my career along what I felt to be the wisest lines. She combined in a marvellous way, a sheltering protection while leaving me the liberty of choice in all my actions. As a result I never felt the urge to escape. On the contrary, I welcomed and sought more and more the harbour of her affection, which proved both stimulating and comforting. She had a firm belief in the power of women to bring common sense and practical knowledge into every aspect of life, both national and international. Given time and opportunity, with their natural tendency to conserve, construct, create, in women lay the greatest hope for peace. She was never defeatist in outlook. Hers was a belief in the ultimate power of good over evil, a belief founded not on religion but on the disciplined forces of human beings, especially women, and quite irrespective of class. Life was not given us for self-indulgence, for material gains, but rather to find in the pursuit of happiness that the greatest happiness lay in work achieved.

This was something of the background I could not fail to absorb when I plunged into making what I could out of life. From her side she showed a touching reliance on my common sense advice over many of the time-consuming complications of a hard-working, delicate writer and Sussex landowner. I helped her with many things, including tax returns, which seems to me now a most rash undertaking! Altogether, during intervals in my studies, I acted almost as her ADC. I might have spent too much time on these behests except for the fact that she was constantly away at Rounton (the Hugh Bell's Yorkshire place) and during the years 1914–20 she crossed the Atlantic several times, as well as travelling all over England to lecture for the Food Ministry.

Now after qualification in 1920 the focus shifted. Medicine became 'the jealous mistress who would brook no rival'. I was thirty-three, and my devotion to E.R. became more adult. I felt myself more on equal terms; in fact, over some things I felt a superior knowledge. The years I'd watched her handling of situations and people, her trust in talking to me about many difficult problems, all contributed to give me a sound psychological insight. With my qualification the tone of E.R.'s letters changed. After eight years of struggling to overcome obstacles, I had justified her unflinching faith.

9
A MENTAL HOSPITAL IN
1920:
'Thrown to the Lions'?

I had made up my mind that my next step was to get a House Physician's post at St Mary's. So I went at once and put down my name as a candidate for Sir John Broadbent's post. I was turned down but not discouraged as I had never been on his firm and he knew nothing of my work. What I most wanted was to be House Physician to Dr Wilfred Harris.

I went to dine with the Kettles immediately after I qualified. Pam Kettle had always been my friend and standby. Dr Harold Kidd, Medical Superintendent of Graylingwell Mental Hospital, Chichester, was there. After we'd enjoyed a good meal and were all feeling cheerful, he suddenly said he was looking for a locum assistant. He would like a woman, the pay was good, would I like the job? I was overwhelmed and much tempted, but I'd had no special experience with lunatics. 'Oh they are mostly exactly like ordinary patients,' he smiled, 'though you may be told by one that she is Queen Victoria.' I explained that I was determined to try for Dr Harris's House Physician. Here Dr Kettle came in, 'Nothing to prevent your taking the job temporarily until his post is advertised. In fact Harris might feel he'd like a House Physician with a little mental experience behind her.' I asked if I might think it over. 'Better than that,' replied Dr Kidd, 'come down on Monday and I'll show you the place and you can decide after that. I'll send my car over to Henfield for you.' I hurried back to E.R. 'I've got a job offered me and it's well paid as a locum.' She was thrilled, but doubtful; mental patients – rather grim perhaps and a stiff introduction to medical practice for a sensitive spirit. It is only recently that I have come to know how deep was her horror of mental hospitals. Her mother had been in one for many years and she was haunted by the memory of her visits to her. She did not relish my starting, even as a locum, in such an institution, but she exercised no determined opposition and left me free to choose. She advocated my seeing the place, though she too felt strongly the superior claim of Dr Harris's House Physicianship.

I stayed the night at Graylingwell and was taken round the particular wards which would be my responsibility. I was introduced to the various sisters and some of the patients. I was deeply impressed by Dr Kidd in action – human, kind, full of common sense and obviously beloved by patients and staff alike, and there was a particular atmosphere about the hospital which attracted me. Or was it a picture of William Wilberforce in the hall which finally decided me to accept the post? I returned to Backset full of enthusiasm which I didn't find shared by E.R., but she agreed that it was a wise step for a short while. I went into Brighton to see Dr Martindale who also strongly disapproved, 'much better have had a holiday', and she sent me back discouraged. Probably it was the only time I didn't take her advice. I had given my word.

The morning of my arrival I presented myself at Dr Kidd's office. He shook hands gravely and with no more ado handed me a bunch of keys, told me which wards were my work, showed me out of the office, and told me where I had better begin. I had expected him to accompany and start me off in a ward, at least, but not a bit of it. I felt I was thrown to the lions. I walked down a corridor feeling rather numb. Oh well, this is a challenge, I said to myself, as with beating heart I unlocked the ward door. The sister came to meet me and I found my self-confidence returning as I faced the first patient in bed. I began at once to learn the patients' names, I read their notes and plunged into trying to help them. One wiry muscular lady was in a ward by herself and I was warned by the sister not to visit her alone. She was at times homicidal. She was also a beautiful dancer, as I learned at the Christmas festivities. While I talked to her I considered how best I would defend myself if suddenly attacked! But we never came to grips and, with me, she was always gentle and well behaved.

[Octavia Wilberforce's experience at Graylingwell Mental Hospital is here related through her letters to Elizabeth Robins:]

December 12th 1920

I found your letter after I came in from the terrific do with the Lunacy Commissioner, Dr B. Thank you so much. It was vastly interesting going round with him, and I'm longing to hear his report. He's an acute, very clever little man and didn't ask me anything tiresome, indeed barely spoke to me, so all was well. Dr N. is very decent too and awfully nice to work with; as an example let me tell you one incident. I had to write up a note on a patient (supposed to do six a day) whose talk was obscene to last degree. Now, there's a very definite and concise way of writing about forms of lunacy, and the words have technical meanings a little different from everyday use. So one has to be very careful – 'irrational', 'deluded', are examples. Dr N. said he'd help me over what to put down if I'd tell him in my words what I'd made of patients. Over one I said, 'She was quite mad' – a term that means nothing as regards notes. 'Talked about wild things – your moral character particularly.' 'Oh yes,' says he, and had the grace to blush, which only a decent man would have done. 'You say . . .' and he dictated.

Mrs Tines is being reasonable (for her) today. So I've left her alone. She took her own food. Twenty-four hours starvation out of temper (mental condition really) did for her what I'd decided to do, i.e. relieved the high blood pressure and consequently lessened the congestion in her brain. Isn't Nature in her cures rather wonderful? And food plays a huge part. Half the patients need reducing to make 'em better or well – the other half want building up.

I've got a patient [who is] suicidal every month and between times a victim of asthma. I'm putting my back into latter now. When she's got asthma she's quite sane and a very nice girl – everybody loves her. When she hasn't asthma she's suicidal. I would like to cure her of one or t'other. My main regret at leaving here is that I shan't have time to try any treatment long enough to get her well.

December 13th
I've done my morning round today.
Wards A1 Infirmary.
      B1 Private cases.
      C1 Acute cases.

Sisters amazingly nice folk. Patients all very good. One on introduction said mine was a historical name, another that she used to make cricketing flannels for No. 27 Wilberforce! One smiles and makes absurd remarks with, such is my aim, great politeness. I find I have to reproach those who haven't been good, will do that tomorrow.

I do all the womens' wards at night. Responsible for the whole bally shoot of three hundred at night. They call me up if anybody ill. One died yesterday afternoon. Others expected to die in night. O.W. to be summoned if so. Night work only consists as a whole of dealing with the physically ill – little with the mentally. But soon I'm going to write to Martindale and just tell her how far from lazy this job is. There's a post mortem today of the patient who died of T.B. yesterday.

This place is riddled with jealousy; all, more or less civilly, at odds! From the point of view of administration it's very interesting!

The women patients well enough went out and snowballed with the nurses yesterday morning. What do you think of that? They loved it.

December 16th
Don't think this is a dangerous job – it isn't:
1) Because the sisters and nurses are personally responsible for one's safety.
2) 'Cos I'm fairly suspicious – e.g. one very violent patient yesterday was being good as gold and politely asked me to listen to her heart. O.W. politely refused. Her scheme was

to get one within arm's length otherwise employed, merely to spit in one's face or box one's ears. This is a purely exceptional case and I've since been warned to leave her alone. I only quote it to reassure you that I'm not wholly unfitted for this post. Some idiot might straightway have complied and a scuffle with nurses resulted. This particularly to be avoided. Even a tiny bruise on a patient has to be reported.

December 17th

Such a strenuous day. Dr N.'s gone off to Southsea – Dr Kidd in bed with laryngitis, bronchitis. So I'm doing all the female section and any emergency on male section – Dr N. did his round before he went.

In some wards I believe the nurses think I know quite a lot of medicine – this particularly in my own three wards, A, B and C. This morning it took me from 10.30 to 1.0 to do only those. E1 and E2 and F1 and F2 I did after lunch. Nurses there not sufficiently respectful I think; call me Nurse or Miss Wilberforce, both of which is cheek really, in a non-teaching hospital. If they don't alter, I'll tick 'em off. But A1 sister brings me patients every moment of the round with medical diseases. And C1 sister is also, I think, quite impressed. May be mistaken, but I have that sort of feeling.

One poor old lady, Mrs Church, is *very* miserable. Her daughters are out on the common in the cold, with nothing to eat, and no clothes. The voices keep telling her so. So I talked to her, reassuring her; for a moment she'll believe me and cheer up. The moment I'm gone she relapses. So I've written out a statement saying how warm and comfortable they are. She's to read it, and have it read to her at intervals. But I'm afraid it won't help. My heart bleeds for her worried old face.

Another gave me a lecture on the League of Nations, very good indeed. I'd want no better anywhere – tho' she's rather demented about the lower classes who are the cause of all this evil. She was a governess. Ditto another who is miserable because she feels she's 'had such a happy life and lost it'. Won't read books about Florence, Paris, Rome, because it worries her to think of how happy she'd been there and now how she's lost it. I talked to her for forty minutes, terribly tiring. Encouraging her to read and think about the places and how happy she'd been there, yes, how privileged her memories were. 'Oh, I know a thing of beauty is a joy forever,' she said. Encouraged her to play the piano. Said I'd write for music for her to her home. She's been here sometime so if they've destroyed it I shall curse.

But it is interesting how many of them were governesses. Why should teaching send you dotty? Continual hard work, no future, no ambitions, bad pay, eh? It's the inelastic conservative governesses, I notice, in military families who go off. Also dozens of servants, and good number of folk whose husbands have been unfaithful. There might be much research done. Were slaves ever mad? What about its being mentally unhealthy to be the underdog? Socialism is needed. Any lunatics in Detroit? Yes, some of the housewives, I bet!

Mrs Tines was abusive and bad this morning – refused food. I went there at dinner time – she stormed like blazes. Later, I made the nurses fetch her some food, give her a fork (only a spoon allowed in the ward she's in now) and I talked to her, each time changing the conversation when she tried to break out afresh – about the Isle of Wight, France, travelling, God knows what! She ate well. This place is going to make me a very good conversationalist, and is going to be very strengthening in many ways.

There are two women I can't bear – one a governess so incoherent and babbling that I never know what she's trying to say. She's forty odd, and the most lamentable creature I've ever seen, mentally, morally, physically. Harmless but a wreck.

The other is like a wild animal. Not, thank heaven, in my regular care. She tries to strangle anybody if they aren't careful – dances quite humanly! I never seek intercourse with her, she glares at one like a lion in a cage and has a horrible criminal face. I'm quite conscious of putting on 'de bel courage' when within ten yards of her; when she's up, a nurse has to be by her all the time. In bed, even, this is also usually so. I think the nurses who are allotted to take charge of her are brave women. I'd hate it, tho' I quite realise that the danger adds a certain element of – not exactly sport – but something akin to that. Even I feel on my mettle in her vicinity. What's the psychology?

The great joy of this place is that when I'm not in wards I can go and sit or sleep by the fire and rest my soul in peace. My only slight fault is that I've not been out more than two days – partly weather and partly laziness. I'm trying to cultivate a 'tails up' – proud with oneself-disposition. I have to do it, else I'd fail with patients; because I do it, it reacts on myself.

You take it from me, any danger to a doctor is all my eye (tho' my aim is to be ever observant) but nurses – that's a different matter. When Dr Kidd is up and better, I'm going to have a word with him on 'reform'. There may be trouble, but I'm going to say my say.

December 19th

I'm afraid I wrote rather miserably yesterday – was rather fed up with things in general. Better today. Church, 9.45 – 10.45. O.W. the MO on duty. Then a woman's neck had to be seen to in theatre – carbuncle. The rounds till 1.0 p.m. From 2.30 – 4.30 p.m. testing urines.

Tonight with Dr N. Another patient who is violent made a dash for him. Mrs T. accused him of assaulting the woman and herself joined the fray. First time she has been active like that really. Bad of her. Personally I believe if I were there all the time I could keep her good. But life would be impossible in those circumstances. Tomorrow I shall have to treat her medically as well as mentally. 5.45. Mrs Kidd comes in about the dance on 31st, and stayed till 7 p.m. O.W. dropping.

Did I tell you of the patients' dances? Every week, 5.30–6.45. Excellent for them and they love it. I watched for a few minutes and felt quite wretched – the waste, the pity of those lives who are so nearly sane. Or rather, those patients who are at times so perfectly rational – it may be only a few minutes – but it's all so very heartrending.

By the way, by the time I leave here I shall probably have made many enemies. Why? 'Cos I'm a sight more useful in some ways at noticing nurses' schemes than men are. One sister, B1 ward, name of H, is a rotter. I'm determined she's to be taught better while I'm here. My wish is for every patient to get out as much as possible, and to be as happy as possible. B1 ward has not been made a parade ground for her to show off and feel superior in. She's a slacker and I'm all out to take her down. O.W. no fool at doing that. She's obstructive and doesn't want to put herself out. But the sisters who are experienced in *medical* work, as well as mental, are getting mighty polite and helpful.

Incidents in the kitchen, too, haven't escaped me – tho' they did the Commissioner. If they pay me £6.6.0d weekly they shall get their money's worth in criticism. By all of which you'll realise that my sore throat is being worked out on others!

December 20th

Had to break to Dr Kidd that I go on January 1st. He was far too nice about it, as he thinks I'm useful and quite good at the job.

Wasted three quarters of an hour this morning over Mrs Tines, standing over her while she undressed herself quietly and got into bed. Sheer compulsion of will on my part and strangely fatiguing. Tonight I can't describe to you how tiresome she was. Calling me a whore and a prostitute incidentally, too. A question of her taking some medicine was the starting point. She'll have it tomorrow thro' a tube, and after a good reducing as a result (her brain is congested and she needs strong measures to relieve it) she'll be a different being.

It is interesting, isn't it, that women use worse language and are more obscene than men? Why? 'Cos they've been taught to repress it always.

9.30 a.m. Tuesday
Those good N's. Sent me to bed with hot milk at 8.30 last night. Dr N. did my round for me. She brought me hot milk in bed. Result – throat not so painful this morning. They are nice people, as well as good to work with. Must go now. Mrs Tines and Tube. Drat her!

December 22nd
I borrowed a bicycle today and firmly went to Chichester. I may get blown up tomorrow for not staying in to see patients' relatives (visiting day) but today is first day I've been outside the grounds. First day I've been out of house since I can't remember when. Bold bid for liberty. And all the better for it. Cold heaps better – practically gone.

I feel happier again now. Mrs Tines is a wicked old soul, and so much enjoyed having her medicine by tube that she laughed and wants it again. She won't of course! She said she'd known Suffragists who'd been fed by tube 'for a craze', so she'd certainly stand it 'for the fun of the fair'! She's seventy-one and one can't but admire her defiant spirit, but the nurses do have a time with her. Tube feeding very skilfully done and quite pleasant in a place like this.

Another patient – sad case – youngish and of course a governess, I took by the arm and walked halfway round garden this morning. She sits down when nurses try to move her. Having started her off, 'Now, Beatrice, you've got to keep on and walk straight round,' I left her. She went on, only about one mile per hour, but she went on, and sister was thoroughly surprised! I'd be quite good at this job if I stayed long. And I quite like it. Gives you masses of self-confidence. But the chronic cases are the ones who make my heart bleed. So much better if they could be electrocuted – I mean the ones with syphilis who never get well.

December 23rd
Mrs Tines came to herself today.
First, rebellious, abusive, obscene.
Second, ordered into a padded room.

Third, defiant to O.W. in same.

Fourth, O.W. went away and five minutes later, 'Dr W – Dr W', and there was nothing she wouldn't promise to do if she might be allowed back in B1 ward. Since everybody from Dr Kidd downwards has been imploring her to do this for the past several days, she might have come to a little earlier. She has been posing lately, and the few minutes in the padded room were just enough to make her natural. I really thought she was having certain 'symptoms' but she quite took me in. She's a wicked old fiend, but awfully amusing. Must go now, and play badminton!

Christmas Eve, 1920

Dr Kidd came and called on me this morning in my sitting-room. Talked an hour. He's a great infant but a really delightful man. I've much affection for him. Said very polite things about my going. Wished I could have stayed. One or two reforms I'd suggested he raised every conceivable objection to yesterday in Office. Talked quite ten minutes against my suggestions, setting forth all the difficulties. It was a matter of distribution of staff [an extra nurse] at night and I knew the Matron could do better if she chose. After the ten minutes' objections, he suddenly smiled and turned to me: 'But, you know, really I quite agree with you. And the present arrangement is dangerous' (I hadn't urged this side for the nurses at all!) 'and can be managed differently. I'll see Miss C. about it now.'

This afternoon I walked to Chichester to get some sweets for all of us to give the sisters. Joined by Harry and Frank Kidd (16 and 15). Frank says, 'I'm so sorry you're going, just when you were getting really useful.' That means of course that Dr Kidd had mentioned to his family that I was shaping well. And is the best form of testimonial.

The first week I used to be just a little careful in wards. Now, I've no nerves at all and can make pretty well every patient do what I want. Mrs Tines apologised to the nth to me. It's the nurses she ought to apologise to really, but Dr

Kidd was much pleased that I'd got her to do that to me. I believe he imagines my feelings might be hurt!

Christmas Day 1920

Do you know that I've never had a more strange and more proud and in many ways enjoyable day than this. Very largely because it's work, and one's being useful and one's being paid for it. Hang it all, but it does make a difference that one has, after all these years, got to a place where one's really doing something.

7.20 a.m. called.

7.45 dressed, and opened letters.

8.00 Early Service.

9.00 Breakfast.

9.45 Church.

10.45–12.15 Round all wards [with Dr Kidd's family and even his house party], shaking hands with patients and staff and wishing Merry Christmas. I think I did this about 500 times.

12.30. I put feet up, racking headache and sore throat. Small wonder!

1.00 p.m. Lunch.

2.00 p.m. To Dr Kidd's. Children's Christmas tree (was given a calendar and book with great kindness).

3.00 p.m. Played golf on the cricket field, joined by Harry and Frank Kidd.

4.30 p.m. Tea with N's.

5.15 p.m. Kitchen and laundry party.

7.00 p.m. Dinner party at Dr Kidd's.

After dinner, staff dance.

Night round and bed.

What do you think of that for a Merry Christmas? And, as I say, I'm really enjoying the thing. Says Dr Kidd, on my doing the formula with Miss H., the homicidal animal who tries to strangle one if given half a chance, 'I do congratulate you on that. A real improvement.' 'Cos why? She shook hands and smiled and looked humanly at me. It's an amazing thing, but the most lost and hopeless creatures have hidden

away in them something which reacts to Christmas, tho'
nothing else can get a spark of memory or intelligence.
Doesn't that give you a feeling of wonder and surprise? It
melts me a lot.

The only trouble about a place like this is that one feels
one wants to give presents to some of the sisters, but one
mustn't favouritise and one can't give them all presents. Too
many of 'em altogether. I wish you could have been here
today and seen all our doings. Seen too, the huge amount of
courtesy as well as kindliness with which I, and other medical
officers, have been treated. If I died tonight you'd know that
I'd, to some extent, justified my existence, and you'd be
proud, eh?

December 27th

You know, this is an amazingly humanly run place. The
concert, done by staff, quite first-class amateurs. Dr Kidd
said to me one morning, 'I always like to get some of my
nurses from Wales, such good voices.' About four hundred
patients seated in this quite beautiful hall, fine stage and
orchestra at end; gallery at t'other end, where medical officers
and stray friends sit. Men patients one side of middle
gangway, women t'other. About a dozen nurses sprinkled in
among the women patients, male attendants among the men.
Staging, limelight, footlights, curtain on same model, tho'
smaller, as a London stage.

The carols they sang in darkness. Men in old caps and
turned-up collared coats. Women in cloaks with hoods and
oil lanterns. Snow falling. Extraordinarily well staged and
well done. Dr Kidd and I descended into the throng at one
juncture. In back row on men's side were a man and woman
sitting affectionately together. Against all rules, theoretically,
really for this to happen. They were brother and sister.
Music? A patient played! She's a harmless imbecile, has to
be led about and ordered what to do, weeps copiously if
spoken to, more or less. But has this gift. It is interesting
here, you know. And one does get really attached to some
of the patients.

December 28th

Today, so far, has been a real red letter one. Dr N. has gone off for the night and I'm in charge. Terribly set up.

I've done quite good spade work here for any future woman who might like to come. One of the sisters (whom I don't care for at all) was awfully sorry to hear I was going, and frankly felt I'd be a real loss. Before I came they were all very agitated and hated the thought of a woman doctor. I can only tell you the following to show you a little of the impression I've made.

Sister P. of A1 ward, and Sister W. of C1., both have picked out nurses for me to look at, and prescribe for. Observe, that's a huge tribute. Sister K. of E1. has often said, 'Oh, Dr N. wants you to look at this patient, please.' – patients he's puzzled over diagnosis. And when I forgot she'd remind me and not let me off. And she'd pick out patients herself for me to tackle – difficult ones. Sister W. of C1. – the noisy, troublesome ward – always would rake up one or two patients to be patched up.

Sister W. has a party for the patients on Wednesday. 'I hardly like to ask you, doctor, because ours is such a rowdy ward and we can't settle down to any great amusement like the other wards; but it would be nice if you could look in on our party, if only for a short while.' Of course I will. These sisters get up the party, supply a lot of the gay parts of the food, and all the amusements and games themselves. Don't you think it's rather splendid? I do. They shall certainly have every encouragement. Dr Kidd thanked me about sharing in Christmas festivities, 'You might have been an old medical officer.' A tribute.

I'm left today and tomorrow in charge of both male and female wards. Further, tomorrow is visiting committee day and I'll probably have to take round a couple of County Councillors, who only come to pry and pick holes if they can. This, too, shows the confidence placed in O.W. I hate having to show the patients and talk about them.

December 30th, 1920

8.50.a.m. This before breakfast.

I want to say that this time here has been the best thing that could have happened to me. And I honestly can't remember enjoying myself more, ever. This I say because always previously enjoyment has not entailed responsibility and the sense of doing real service to chunks of people. Don't think I'm being priggish about it, but this is the honest truth and I've never in all my born days been so set up.

Dr N. went off Monday 9.45 a.m., returned 5.30 p.m. yesterday, Tuesday. During that time I carried on the male side as well as this. And never have my legs felt so inclined to ache, if they'd had time to realise it, but they didn't! It was hard work. And one or two men badly ill; and a male admission, and two members of County Council visiting, to take round. Everybody, I think, pleased with O.W.'s work. O.W. pleased too.

There is an ex-service man who uses the most awful language and is very violent. I was warned about him. He began as soon as I entered the ward. I *stopped* that man, and he talked to me quite more or less civilly. The attendants can't stop him, he goes on with them all day. Another spits in your face by way of playing up (he's a Rumanian). I didn't know till after which he was. And I bent right over him and asked about the book he was reading. I noticed attendants rather restive but all went happily.

Monday night Sister P. gave a 'patients' party'. That means she supplies extra cakes, jellies, nuts, oranges, no small matter as there are sixty people at it. First a huge feed, 4–5 p.m. Then musical chairs and dancing, games till 8.45. Part of my job to go. Dr Kidd thanks you for doing that! But I've never enjoyed any party so much. Why? 1) I enjoy the dancing. 2) The patients enter into it and the worst of 'em become human, light-hearted and gay. The sad ones throw away their depressions, the ones who hear voices aren't troubled by them, the violent ones throw themselves and their energy into enjoying themselves.

After breakfast

Last night there were two parties, O.W. terribly torn to keep the balance. Sister W. in C1 – the acute ward. Can't hear yourself speak, and patients liable to hit each other (or nurses) in the face all day. But bless you, they are blindfolded in turn and draw the pig's tail on the floor; they play musical chairs; they dance; and their language has all the bad words omitted, and they forget that voices tell 'em this and that; and they don't quarrel; and they love it.

After dinner, I'd asked Sisters P. and K., the two senior sisters, to come and see me. And many civilities passed. They were so sorry I was leaving so soon (tho' they'd been rather against my coming). I say what I think of how they work. People are too beastly chary of appreciation in this life.

Yesterday, a field day.

Male wards from 10–12, female wards from 12–1.

Female wards with visiting committee, 2.15–3.15

Male wards with visiting committee, 3.15–4.15

Male admission, 4.15–4.30

Seeing patients' relatives, 4.30–4.45

Writing up weekly journal, 4.45–4.50

Not being able to finish then, I continue from 8.15–8.30 p.m.

Hasty tea, 4.50–5.0

C1 party, 5.0–6.0

E1 party, 6.0–7.10

My, but it was a day.

The visiting committee so boring. Asking stupid questions, but you see how I've picked up the work and do all that Dr N. does when he's here. And just to keep 'em up to the mark, I'll inspect the medicine cupboards in the wards. If I find untidiness, and medicines and lotions on same shelf (danger in that) there'll be trouble. Or rather, not trouble, 'cos I don't believe in being cross with people, but firm and reasonable. And the sisters here, from what I can see of them, are quite exceptionally open to reason.

Thank you so much for your most understanding letters.

133

It makes the whole difference – makes one put one's back into it twice over.

When I left Graylingwell on 31 December 1920 I was inordinately proud of my first earned professional cheque and I was deeply moved at leaving. I had loved my time there, and it certainly benefited my work. [My experience there] early taught me that the body can be more receptive to treatment than the mind, although in countless patients these two factors are interwoven in a manner frequently impossible to disentangle. It had also given me a self-confidence and grasp which no other job could have done in so short a time. When I left Dr Kidd wrote me a heartening and encouraging letter.

On 16 December I [had] heard I had been chosen for Dr Harris's House Physician post, without even the ordeal of an interview. I had been lucky as my opponent was academically a strong candidate and I feared he would have had the job. But he had not been a Clinical Clerk on Dr Harris's firm whereas Dr Harris did know me. [After my Graylingwell experience] I started off at St Mary's Hospital on 1 January 1921 full of confidence and enthusiasm. This was my first job of real responsibility.

10

FIRST HOSPITAL POSTS IN LONDON

1921–22

1921 was a critical period in the annals of St Mary's Hospital. In the hospital world medical teaching was being reorganised and four teaching hospitals in London had been given university grants to start medical and surgical units. There was only enough money for one more and the decision had to be made as to which hospital was the best for teaching purposes. Top-level discussions took place and we were inspected by an impressive little band of advisers, chosen from the consultants of other hospitals. Dr Wilson (now Lord Moran), who was indefatigable in his work for St Mary's, was indomitably active in pushing forward our claims. Finally it was arranged that we should be put on probation for six months and then it would be decided whether St Mary's Hospital or our rival should obtain fifth place.

Professor Pannett was more than ready to be the surgical professor but the medical side was more difficult. Dr Wilfred Harris, who was primarily a brilliant neurologist, was induced to act as head of the Medical unit for six months with Dr Wilson as the Assistant Director. It was immense luck for me that when the appointment of House Physician was made, Dr Harris chose me at this critical time. Dr Harris was a first-class physician and instead of concentrating on pure Neurology he was, at this period, compelled to teach General Medicine.

My first weeks at St Mary's Hospital needed all my newly won assurance. I was confronted by a number of clinical clerks of both sexes who had to write up the cases adequately and I had to learn which could be relied on to do this before Dr Harris's round. I had to absorb all the details about the patients who had been in the ward before I took over, and I made a horrid mistake over a new admission. A man was sent in for an injection for trigeminal neuralgia, the procedure for which Dr Harris was world-famed. These cases generally came in for only one night. It was January and there was a great call on beds for pneumonias and other urgencies. The sooner he was dealt with and the bed released the better, so I rang up Dr Harris and asked him to come along and deal with the case. All the paraphernalia for injection was ready waiting on the trolley for the great man. He arrived, with his throat muffled up, nearly speechless with laryngitis, stalked up to the patient and began to examine him. Then he turned round and eyed me, with contempt and rage: 'Have you examined this case, Miss Wilberforce?'

'No sir. As he was only sent in for injection,' I began.

But he cut me short: 'Then you'd better,' in withering tones. 'He's not a trigeminal at all – getting me up out of bed on a wild goose chase.' He turned to Sister Albert, who immediately sympathised over his throat, and I stammeringly apologised. I felt utterly miserable and a complete fool. My God, what a beginning! Completely crestfallen, I accompanied him in silence back through the ward and down the stone stairs along the corridor which seemed endless on that occasion. 'More things are missed by not looking than not knowing,' he growled in the blackest of moods. I assured him that I'd *never* be so remiss again and he suddenly turned, smiled quite humanly, and said goodbye in a forgiven-this-time tone which I felt I had certainly not deserved. Needless to say, he never again saw a patient during my term of service that I hadn't examined with every atom of care at my command!

Shortly after this unfortunate incident I was going round Albert Ward with Sister. 'Why has this poor chap been all this time running a septic type of temperature, Sister?' I was told he had been at first suspected of having an acute infective endocarditis, but this was not the case. He had no sign of tuberculosis and he was still undiagnosed, but there was no doubt he was going downhill, and Sister was worried. I read his notes again and questioned him as to his history. This gave me an idea. I went over him carefully and at last found a deep-seated lump in his back. I was thrilled. 'I believe he has a perinephric abscess,' I told Dr Harris on his next visit. He was impressed, re-examined him, agreed with my diagnosis and asked Professor Pannett to operate. A week later another man came in who had been ill quite a while and was running a septic type of temperature. Nobody had diagnosed him. Now a perinephric abscess is not a common affliction; in fact I had never seen one before, but I diagnosed the same thing. As he seemed very ill, I asked Mr Bryan, whose day it was for surgical emergencies, to see him. He agreed with the diagnosis and operated at once. Full of my own brilliance I reported this to my Chief next day. He was very angry indeed. Why hadn't I asked *him* to see the case before referring it to a surgeon? Suppose it had proved to be something different? After all the man was sent in for his opinion. I apologised and said I would never do it again. He forgave me and finally suggested I should write up these two unusual cases for the *Lancet* and, if I liked, he would add a note. I told Pam [Kettle], who was delighted, and my 'beginner's luck' earned me quite a flash-in-the-pan reputation. The *Lancet* published my report and I subsequently received a letter from a doctor in Czechoslovakia who was making a study of perinephric abscess.

I soon found out that being a House Physician was a responsible job and I loved every minute in spite of many anxious moments. It was a stimulating and valuable experience to work under Dr Harris. He expected the best from his House Physician and realised he could trust me to tell him the truth rather than save my skin by a lie. He was gentle and kind, as a rule, with the patients, though he easily saw through any malingering. One slim, dark, pretty girl was brought in to Medical Casualty unconscious. She had several abdominal scars and could not be roused. I tried every means at my disposal after I had admitted her and ordered rectal feeds to keep her alive. Her temperature and pulse were both within normal limits and there were no positive signs to give one a lead. Dr Harris then examined and tested her and again there was no response. But with a wicked grin at me he suddenly made a very rude remark about the girl's looks. There was an immediate flicker of her eye-lashes! 'Don't worry. She's all right.' Hysteria. We soon got her up and ready to go out. This girl had a devotion to hospitals and her scars were due to various unnecessary operations at other hospitals where she had successfully taken in some unwary young surgeons. About a year later, when I was Assistant Medical Officer at Paddington Infirmary, I was roused from my bed to see a desperately ill young woman – 'query cerebral tumour' – completely unconscious, brought in by the police. I recognised this girl at once, ordered her a hot bath, and reassured the police by saying we'd take her in for a few nights, but it was only hysteria. At this, one of the policemen in amazement said, 'Do you know, I believe I remember taking her in to the Middlesex some months back. She evidently enjoys hospital life, a cheap way of living that wouldn't appeal to me!' We couldn't trace any relatives, but it is not likely that she gave her real name. When not 'enjoying hospital life' it was presumed she lived on the streets.

The sitting-room allotted to generations of Dr Harris's House Physicians was not particularly cheerful. It had a hard horse-hair couch, a table and two or three chairs, but it meant a lot to me. As I was never short of flowers, either from Backset or grateful patients, its bareness could be mitigated and after a time the threadbare carpet was replaced. At different times various friends were asked to tea and were, I hoped, suitably impressed when the porter summoned me to attend an emergency, as was always liable to happen. My visitors included Sir Hugh Bell, Mrs Yates Thompson, Aunt Betty Milbank, and even my mother, on one occasion, to see for herself what I was up to. E.R., of course, came many times; I had the Wilsons (now Morans) to meet her and they became her friends too. They were always particularly kind to me.

I was nearly at the end of my House Physicianship [when I was summoned urgently to the Dean (Dr Wilson)]. I hurriedly looked at the patients in the wards who were giving me anxiety and, promising to return to finish my round, I reported to the Dean's office. He asked me what my next move was to be and suggested I should put in for the position of Assistant Medical

Officer at Paddington Infirmary, Harrow Road. The appointment was to be made shortly and the application ought to be
in by Wednesday. There was no time to be lost. It was good
pay and under the new arrangement the Infirmary would be
ancillary for teaching purposes to St Mary's Hospital. He would
be the consultant on the medical side, Professor Pannett on the
surgical side and he thought I would be the right person for
the job. He'd always be willing to help me, would teach on
selected cases twice weekly, and I should have clinical clerks
under me from St Mary's Hospital. I did not really fancy the
job, nor the thought of having only to deal with a lot of 'old
chronics'. Dr Wilson saw my reluctance to take the post and
urged me to go up and see Miss Morris who was in charge of
the obstetrics and medical beds, and bargain with her to let me
have some of her 'acute' beds. They were extremely good cases
and often not so desperately ill as the ones sent in to a teaching
hospital; in fact, urged the Dean, they were more like the
majority of cases in general practice. I had to get some testimonials and there were only two days. Dr Wilson mentioned a
promising male rival who was up for the job and was persuasive
against my reluctance. I consulted Dr Wilfred Harris, who said
it was an excellent idea and would give me the self-reliance I
needed to be on my own in a responsible post.

I went up to see Miss Morris and was horrified at the closeness of the beds on the bare scrubbed boards and the general
bleakness of the wards. Miss Morris was co-operative, would
prefer me to a man, and after negotiations agreed to exchange
the care of some acute beds for chronic ones if the Medical
Superintendent, Dr Stewart, agreed. She stipulated she would
keep all the obstetric beds. I'd have to teach students from St
Mary's and pick out good cases for Dr Wilson for teaching on
his bi-weekly rounds. I went back to St Mary's terribly torn.
Perhaps it would be useful for general practice and it would be
nice to earn something, as the House Physician's job was not
paid. Lord Buxton was very generously still allowing me £50
for the first six months after qualification, but this was due to
end. The alternative was to try for the Medical Registrarship at
St Mary's and in time, I hoped, get my membership. I'd been

very happy during the last six months over my clinical work, but I did long to specialise in General Medicine. Finally I consulted my kind friend, Pam Kettle. She and Professor Kettle were absolutely confident that I would do well in the future, for he had apparently kept an eye, as pathologists often do, on my House Physician's work. He offered to write a testimonial to help me get the post if I did put in for it. By the time I'd also got testimonials from Dr Harris and Professor Pannett (each so laudatory that they made me blush), and rushed up to deliver them at the eleventh hour at Paddington Hospital, I was immensely keen about getting that job.

The interview was truly alarming. There were a number of Guardians as well as Dr Stewart, the Medical Superintendent, who had already interviewed me when I saw Miss Morris. I was asked 'What was my ultimate aim?' I said firmly, 'general practice'. They then asked some quite irrelevant questions which I did my best to answer. Then I retired to wait with the other candidate who was very bright, had better qualifications and, I felt sure, would be chosen. They kept us waiting quite a long while but finally I was summoned. They were happy to appoint me. I hurried back to St Mary's Hospital, told Sister Albert and wired to E.R. A princely salary of one pound a day. I felt rich indeed.

I can never regret the time spent at Paddington Hospital which taught me many things. At St Mary's Hospital most of the patients sent for admission were advanced cases of serious illness. The Paddington Hospital clientele proved to be more in the earlier stages. There were many more patients directly under my care, but it was easier to reach a stage of intimacy when they would confidentially disclose clues about their life which could help in diagnosis. One patient was a stalwart Scottish dock labourer who had a solid effusion of blood under his skin on the outer side of one leg from his hip to his heel. He denied any fall or injury, was unmarried and earned a good wage, which he told me proudly he spent on buying the good food he cooked himself. His general practitioner, a specialist and myself were all at a loss for a diagnosis. Blood disease was suspected but the routine blood examination cancelled this out.

One day [the dour Scot and I] found a common interest and had a long talk on the art of cooking, in which I was always interested, and he enlarged on the way he cooked his beefsteaks. 'The best you can buy,' he kept repeating.

'What do you eat with it?' I asked.

'Bread and a good cup of tea.'

'No vegetables, no greens, no fruit or tomatoes or salad?' His excellent beef twice a day, he stoutly maintained, was enough. He spent about two pounds or more a week on it. I thought I'd found the answer and couldn't wait for the next visit of the pathologist, Dr E.C.J. Calvert, to do a platelet count. He was greatly interested and sure enough the test proved that this man, as I suspected, had scurvy. We plunged in and stretched the resources of the hospital kitchen over demands for salads, fruit, spinach and other greens. Days went by and suddenly his leg began to show all the shades of a rainbow – it was most dramatic. He objected at first 'to being fed like a rabbit', but finally submitted and became greatly intrigued as he watched his skin change back to normal. It was Dr Richard Cabot who, when asked which he thought the more important as an aid to diagnosis in the investigation of a patient, the physical signs or the history, replied that if he was forced to choose only the one method, he would always select a good history.

Early in 1922 I was beginning to feel I knew something of Medicine and that I ought to plan for the future, but it was difficult to decide on my next step. I longed to become a consultant but this meant I must get my MRCP and be a medical registrar while working for it. I would have to find somewhere in London to live and hope to attract a few patients sent by my contemporaries who needed a medical opinion. The honorarium of Medical Registrar at St Mary's Hospital was in those days £100 a year. One could earn a little by coaching students for their medical examinations (in fact I was already doing this in a modest way). But though I was saving up nearly every penny I could earn, it was a step which was certainly risky. I had been lucky as a student in not getting into debt and my determination was to be self-supporting and a burden on no one. My love of Medicine was increasing every day and I was more than anxious to convince my family of my success.

The alternative suggestion was to find a flat in Brighton, put up a plate, and start in general practice, hoping to be a clinical assistant at the New Sussex Hospital, and perhaps in course of time to gain a hospital appointment there; it was one of only three hospitals in England staffed by medical women. The advantages would be that I felt I'd get on with Sussex patients as I myself was Sussex to the core, that I already knew a few people in Brighton, that it would be only ten miles from Backset and from E.R., and there was the lure of roses and even, possibly, golf. The great advantage of London was that I could keep in touch with my medical friends and chiefs and I would continue to have the benefit of Sister Albert's long-experienced and ever vigilant clinical eye.

We all talked endlessly of the next step. Among my friends was Miss Esther Rickards, who was a first-rate surgeon and had made Surgical Registrar at St Mary's Hospital, which showed how highly her work was valued in spite of her outspoken statements championing Labour. She had a remarkable brain, was a beautiful operator, and was inevitably of consultant timber. One day she came to me with a wonderful idea. She had operated on a film actress and looked after her for weeks, and this girl had developed a doglike devotion for Miss Rickards and was inordinately grateful. She was only twenty-one and had inherited a fortune of £1000 a year from her Russian mother. She wanted to buy 64 Harley Street for Miss Rickards to set up there, and Miss Rickards would like me and E.R. to join her and have an upper flat, and I could have patients there while being Medical Registrar. I immediately wrote to E.R. and got her to come and look at the house and meet Miss Rickards and the girl, who was a small, gentle, attractive creature, who only looked about seventeen. Everything seemed a Great Adventure and we were all thrilled by the prospect. There were nice big rooms for E.R. and the house was in good condition. My future seemed settled. We made every sort of plan.

On 16 May the bubble had burst. The film star had suddenly

disappeared and all her tales were a pack of lies! This was shattering news and all my plans had to be reconsidered. I had spent several weeks envisaging my future as Medical Registrar at St Mary's. Now I had to think again. The future of Backset was at this time in the balance, for E.R. was anxious to migrate to London to keep more in touch with her friends. E.R. resolved to keep Backset as headquarters, but she would try to let this haven of peace, and meanwhile it was important to find caretakers. After I had interviewed for her a promising secretary/housekeeper to take charge, E.R. wrote:

What you forget is that you *can't* put energy and time into service for Backset for these next years – your energy and time have got to go into your profession. Backset must give you recreation, good air, and peace (might incidentally give you eggs).

Where we women fail is in not wisely deputing. You and I would not lose, but gain, if we made a better investment of Backset. I have blamed myself for letting you do too much there. Your strength and wits are needed for things other people can't do at all. At the same time Backset 'service' is a highly important factor in our two lives.

At the hospital I was at cross-purposes with a new Medical Superintendent who was not of the same calibre as his predecessor. I was not alone in thinking that he was not putting his back into the job sufficiently, but being possibly the oldest Assistant Medical Officer, I was deputed to tackle him about his slackness, which was hampering the medical care of patients. Very naturally he was furious, and Dr Wilson had to intervene.

There is no doubt I was restless and anxious to get settled. It looked as if Brighton might after all be the solution. E.R. was constantly going down to Board of Management meetings of the New Sussex Hospital and returned one day with the news that Dr Martindale had sold her practice and was to make London her centre. This news depressed me utterly, for one of the attractions of Brighton was the fact that she would be there and might possibly help me with advice and introductions. It was a great blow, but I felt the usefulness of Paddington was coming to an end and there were many frustrations.

One specially warm summer's day a patient died and I particularly wanted a post-mortem to examine certain organs which had been responsible for the death. This was a job that couldn't be postponed because of the hot weather. I'd watched Dr Spilsbury and Dr Kettle do many post-mortems and knew the procedure all right so I decided to do it myself. But I had not reckoned on the need for practice. It took me over four hours to complete that examination and I don't remember ever sweating more copiously. I was encased in heavy rubber aprons and gloves and had no assistant to help me. The sweat poured into my eyes and I couldn't wipe my face with bloody hands. I resolved I would not tackle another autopsy, though Dr Phillips always said that the post-mortem room was where one learnt most Medicine.

The summer at Paddington provided interesting work, but I had a good deal of anxiety about E.R.'s health, the future of Backset, my own future, and a feeling of pressure that time was marching on. I was then thirty-four and I ought to be free and capable of taking up medical practice on my own. I was desperately tired for it was a specially hot summer and there was a bad epidemic of infantile diarrhoea. The whole staff and the nurses were rushed off their feet. Mothers were bringing in babies day and night, nearly moribund, and it was heartbreaking how little one could do for them.

Always faithful and responsive to spas, E.R. went to Saltsjobaden in Sweden during July, where she had treatment which was helpful, but she decided she would like to return via Freiburg for further medical counsel. Then the Bells intervened and pointed out the folly of such a step [in view of] the disastrous further fall of the mark [and Germany's political situation]. Wouldn't E.R. instead come to Rounton and bring me too? So this was done and my holiday was spent learning to drive a motor. Surprisingly enough this was at Maurice Bell's suggestion. I say surprisingly because he was rather deaf, and struck me as an unhappy man in both his home surroundings and his work. But being told I would probably go into practice in

Brighton, he had the imagination to say I must certainly have a car and could I drive? Sir Hugh's efficient chauffeur, George White, taught me on a huge, heavy Crossley, but before I left I was allowed to drive Maurice's Daimler. Those were the days of double declutching, and I think it was trusting of them to allow a novice to risk damaging the gears.

One other experience restored any slight lessening of morale. The local doctor, who was a delightful man, while paying medical visits at Rounton had been introduced to me. He took my breath away by asking me if I would come and see a lad he was deeply concerned about: 'Perhaps, sometimes, a fresh mind might be helpful,' he courteously and rather diffidently suggested. I was thrilled, flattered and much interested in the case for which he was doing everything possible. The only help I was capable of giving was to make the same diagnosis and boost his morale. When specially worried over a desperately ill patient, it is always a particular relief to have another mind to go into the case. This holiday in the brisk Yorkshire air, playing tennis and driving around the countryside, was a delightful rest and adventure and I returned to London full of new hope for the future.

11

PUTTING UP A PLATE IN BRIGHTON

General Practice

1923–40

After the collapse of the Harley Street Bubble and a summer of indecision, I finally decided that Brighton was to be my fate. I began to look for a flat or a maisonette but I could find nothing. At last I saw 24 Montpelier Crescent. It was near the hospital and near the station and the cost was £3000. By comparison with horrible flats at exorbitant rentals it seemed a good risk, but how could I raise the capital? I applied to each of my married sisters who had rich husbands. I had saved, since qualification, just over £300 myself, but after negotiation the house would cost £2900. Miss Robins spoke to Mrs Yates Thompson, who promptly said she had left me £1500 in her will, and would give it now. I tried hard to think of somebody I knew who would lend me the rest of the money. Finally I approached Trudie Lady Denman. She had married my first cousin and I knew [she] believed in women's work. She at once asked, 'Why not tackle your rich sisters?'

'I have, but neither will help!'

'Slunges,' she replied with emphasis, and lit another cigarette. She asked me many searching questions – and appreciated the fact that if I could get a foot in at the New Sussex Hospital – which she generously supported – it would help me greatly. 'I'll lend you £1200,' she suddenly exclaimed, and she smiled enchantingly as she made a few uncomplimentary remarks about my relatives. I flushed and stammered my thanks but she cut me short and took me to the door. I staggered out into Upper Grosvenor Street not able to believe my good fortune.

146

But E.R. was thoroughly worried. She hated the thought of my starting heavily in debt. She herself had started on a loan of $500 and knew what the burden of a loan can be. All the same, though disapproving, she was most co-operative, and came to realise that 24 Montpelier Crescent was not so bad an investment. I took the plunge and bought the house. Early in January 1923 I moved into 24 Montpelier Crescent and put up my brass plate.

Dr Wilson had cheered me greatly when, with a most laudatory testimonial, he enclosed a private note:

I must tell you how grateful I am for all you have done at the Infirmary to make the teaching a going concern. It has been very pleasant to work with you and what you did went a long way to make the classes and clerking go.

I hope Brighton may be a great success. I have no doubt whatever it will be. There must inevitably be times of discouragement but in the end all will come out right. We all tend to be over anxious about the mere business of making money. In reality the rewards of practice are of a different kind and you will find that they go far to mitigate the worry inseparable from an uncertain art.

During the first weeks in my new home I slipped on the newly varnished floor and yet again dislocated the cartilage of my knee which resulted in synovitis. This meant enforced rest and I had to retire to bed. During this time Dorothy Wilson paid me a visit which enormously heartened me. She told me that to have an accident on entering a new house was a portent of good luck to follow! It was more than consoling as I lay upstairs, thinking of the shining new brass plate, an invitation to patients to call. The arranging of the furniture [was] still to be done, with the help of a not very intelligent servant. The brass plate proved depressingly unco-operative in its appeal for several weeks, but I had Clinical Assistant work at the hospital, and I also gave anaesthetics, so that I wasn't idle. Dr Martindale had told me that I must at once go and call on the medical practitioners in the town, and this I presently did. The doctors

I called on were civil, especially the consultants, though all were perhaps a little doubtful about my wisdom in 'putting up a plate'. As I look back, it certainly was a risk.

I worked hard as Clinical Assistant to Outpatients at the New Sussex Hospital and after a time found that I was occasionally sent for by the mistresses of the maids I had helped in Outpatients. It was a nucleus and in course of time began to enlarge. In my first year from April 1923 to 1924 I earned £308.

There are times in a doctor's life when frustrations and the domestic problems of a patient's life make one despair of being adequately helpful. This was where occasional visits to Mrs Yates Thompson had unexpected results, [for she was] a modest, sensitive, wonderful friend. She had a cheerful, light touch which always diverted me. In a mood of great depression, instead of catching an early train home, I had called one evening at Mrs Yates Thompson's and was persuaded to stay to dinner – 'Only Mr Wright coming.' So I decided to take the later train. 'Haggy' arrived and I had five minutes alone with him. He asked me how I was getting on, quite obviously expecting a dubious reply. I replied cheerfully, 'On the crest of the wave' – his face fell with a mixture of bewilderment and disappointment. He plainly didn't like to hear it. Haggy was true brother to Sir Almroth Wright of St Mary's Hospital, who was insanely antagonistic to women and all their work.

Later, [he said] patronisingly: 'It must be rather interesting trying to push your way up, isn't it?'

I paused a long time; I couldn't understand quite what he meant but felt he was trying to be beastly. Remembering my hosts, the Yates Thompsons, I finally said, 'Oh, you mean my putting up a plate instead of buying a practice. It *is* interesting. Of course, if you buy a practice you are more limited as it's not generally considered wise to buy a man's practice.' He agreed heartily and I let it sink in. Then, 'But I've a young friend who against advice did do this. In three months she doubled her practice, and now has more men than women patients. The other day she received a deputation from Great Western railwaymen asking that 250 of them should be transferred to her panel, from the man over the way.' The evening's talk stirred me and, restored by antagonism, I lost my depression and became a determined young doctor once more.

I was beginning to be quite confident in my future success when I went down with bronchial influenza [in January 1925] and my cough became asthmatic. After weeks of ordinary care and treatment, I finally consulted my friend Dr Phillips. He sent me to Switzerland, but I was no better. He then was very firm and ordered sunshine; he even threatened me with tuberculosis, which was alarming. E.R. asked if Florida would be wise and he urged it strongly. Raymond Robins, E.R.'s brother, invited us to Chinsegut and generously offered to pay my fare, but I was most reluctant to desert my practice at this early stage. It was a perilously drastic step to be away from January to March 1925, even though kind Dr Marjorie Hubert, whom I had coached in Clinical Medicine, and who had followed in my footsteps at St Mary's, offered to cherish my patients while I was away.

I got back to my practice renewed in mind and body and eager for patients. I was specially glad to be back in time for the big function – a luncheon to Lady Astor – at which she made a typically witty speech before she opened the bazaar for the New Sussex Hospital. All the hospital supporters turned out in force and any rumour that I was away indefinitely through illness was immediately scotched by my healthy sunburned appearance.

During the next four months my practice began to build up. I had been lucky enough to be made Assistant Physician and allowed the use of two beds in the hospital. One of my patients was a girl with acute endocarditis. The secretary said she was a chronic case and must be removed. I fought this and not so long afterwards, as expected, the poor child died. I knew that her heart was an interesting one and I was anxious to have it properly examined. So having obtained permission to do this from her parents, I went up to London to take it to St Mary's Pathological department, where I deposited it for the expert opinion of Professor Kettle.

I then went to Albert Ward to have tea with Sister Albert and Sister Manvers. Suddenly I felt a pain so acute in my abdomen that I collapsed. Everybody was plainly scared out of their wits. The Dean was luckily in the hospital and was quickly summoned and was also puzzled over my condition. I was taken to Alexandra Ward and carefully watched for an hour or two; was there anyone I would like sent for? E.R. at that moment was in Yorkshire but Dr Martindale I knew to be in London and she came along. The pain had subsided but I still felt ghastly – I suppose completely shocked. Mr Gordon Bryan diagnosed a retrocaecal appendix and I was duly operated on, when it was found that I had an embolus in the appendix. I made an uneventful recovery and was more than grateful when I learned that if this collapse had happened in a taxi or train I should probably not have survived. E.R. came down from Rounton for about a week and came and read to me, and later I convalesced with Dr Martindale at her Sussex home. I was soon driving my car again and playing tennis and felt immediately cheered when one day she looked at me and said: 'Well now, Octavia, you certainly aren't neurotic, are you?' Soon I was thankfully back at work.

1927 was a very hot summer, E.R. had not been feeling well, and with her confidence in spas, she went to Bad Elster in Saxony. I accompanied her for part of the time and we became friendly with Dr Von Kittlitz who treated E.R. and ordered her mud baths. I thought I would like to try them too, which I did after consultation with Dr Von Kittlitz, and thoroughly enjoyed them. We both grew much attached to that kind woman and she came to stay with me in Brighton on three occasions. She had a rare, sensitive mind, with great clinical wisdom, and her intuitive grasp of personalities, combined with much sympathy, made her a dear friend. By her second visit Hitler had gained power. Dr Von Kittlitz was a Prussian and she only practised in Bad Elster during the summer season. She had rooms there and was furious when, one day as she came out of the lavatory, she was stopped and warned that she would be reported if she ever again omitted to lift her hand and say 'Heil Hitler!'

On her last visit she was very silent and seemed to have lost her bubbling sense of fun, which was an ingredient she mixed well with sound medicine and a calm, philosophic turn of mind. Phyllis Ponsonby [née Buxton] was staying with me at the same time, as well as E.R., and in her blunt and forthright way Phyllis suddenly asked, 'What do you think of Hitler?' My good German friend flushed, longed to be truthful, but hesitated. We reassured her that anything she said was only heard by us and she could be quite frank. She took a long breath, her eyes filled with tears and she poured out her hatred of Fascism. She had been so conditioned to Gestapo methods that she had never dared speak openly until then. She confessed she still was haunted by the thought that perhaps someone concealed might repeat her talk. She enjoyed her visit and became her old cheerful self again and was a real asset as a guest. She and Phyllis became fast friends – they both valued freedom in speech as well as action. It was with much sorrow that I learned after the end of the war that she was killed by our last raid on Dresden.

Dr Von Kittlitz had entirely won E.R.'s confidence and greatly helped her make decisions for a more settled, comfortable future. Albion Street was an inconvenient house and E.R. eventually moved to 6 Palace Gate, a charming top flat with large rooms and the writing-room of her dreams. Winnie Inglis, a maid who had been for years with the D'Oyley Cartes, contributed much to her comfort there. Brighton served as a bolt hole for weekends, and sometimes when nursing and convalescence became necessary, as E.R.'s health was likely to collapse at intervals after strenuous bouts of London life. She never found it easy to say 'No' to the invitations and demands of her many friends, while she always devoted the mornings and early evenings to her writing. She had a bad attack of thrombophlebitis which worried me greatly and I had her and a nurse at Brighton.

[In 1934 Octavia Wilberforce accompanied E.R. to New York. While E.R. dealt with pressing family and business affairs Octavia pursued her interests in medical research:]

Armed with medical introductions, I went with a letter from Tom Kettle, my pathologist friend, to see Professor Peyton Rous. Professor Kettle had said he was engaged on what might prove epoch-making research. Later I was entertained at lunch at the Rockefeller Institute. Alexis Carrell, the founder of the Carrell Dakin treatment of wounds, showed me his work. Noguchi, the small, keen, poker-faced Japanese, the discoverer of the cause and cure of yellow fever, showed me his specimens. It was tragic that he, years afterwards, died of this fell disease. While we were sitting at lunch a slim, fair-haired, youthful figure slid into the room and seated himself at a table with his back to all the company and looked wistfully out of the window over the Hudson River. 'That,' said my host, 'is Lindbergh. He is doing research here but he shuns publicity and hates anybody to notice him.'

Martha Draper and Dorothea Blagden, both sisters of Ruth Draper, asked me to lunch and I was shown more medical work in hospitals. We also went to Gertrude Stein's *Four Saints in Three Acts*, urged thereto by Dr George Draper. We lunched with Mrs Janie Nicols (Lady Buxton's friend and daughter of J.P. Morgan), and I was impressed when I found that nobody smoked, there were no cocktails and no wine. But the cost of the Plaza! I had gained many medical facts and was melted by the warmth and hospitality of the American friends. We returned on the *Adriatic* and it was an immense relief to get back to medical practice.

A colleague once told me it was important for a successful physician to be a father-confessor as well. It often facilitates a cure or can prevent illness if patients confide their anxieties and worries. That was how Backsettown came to be started. It grew to be more and more clear to me that a patient's anxiety over personal difficulties of all kinds were the contributing, if not the sole cause, of the indigestion, insomnia, irritability which was so hard to control or cure. I was certain that a rest pause could prove a definite piece of preventive Medicine. Had I not in my student days only succeeded in battling through my home frustrations and exam fears by the diversion of rose growing and the happiness and peace I found at Backsettown? E.R. had become more involved in her London activities and was anxious to settle there to see more of her friends. She generously consented, for a small rental, to allow Backsettown to be used as a convalescent home to provide such a rest pause for professional women and tired housewives. We formed a small committee with Phyllis, now Lady Phillis Ponsonby, as our chairman, and Miss Evelyn Fellows, OBE as honorary secretary. Somehow, funds had to be raised, furniture bought and staff secured. Mrs Campion, by this time well on in years, was instrumental in extracting money from many hardened stones and we had a number of useful gifts. We started boldly on an overdraft guaranteed by Phyllis Ponsonby, Lady Leconfield and Sir Richard Denman. The domestic staff was a difficulty. The idea of meals on trays, in garden or bedrooms, was considered revolutionary, and we had no less than seven cooks and six house parlourmaids during our first year.

We made a good beginning, but the slump hit us badly and by 1933 we should have had to close down but for the generosity of Ruth Draper. She flew over from Paris and gave us a matinee at the Theatre Royal when Dame Madge Kendal made a moving appeal. It was a brilliant occasion and Ruth was at her best. The proceeds were equally divided between Backsettown and the New Sussex Hospital. A representative committee of Sussex names worked hard at selling every ticket, but I had all the anxieties of a producer in the more intimate detailed arrangements, and I thoroughly enjoyed it.

After being appointed to the staff of the New Sussex Hospital I was made Secretary to the Medical Committee at a time when Dr Martindale was the Chairman. I suffered agonies over the work since Dr Martindale was a perfectionist and I found it almost impossible to reduce long discussions to sizeable proportions. She instructed me with endless patience and after a time I was elected to the Board of Management of the New Sussex Hospital. In spite of the economic depression this was the period when the hospital was enlarging its activities by rebuilding, increasing the number of beds and the nursing accommodation, appointing a pathologist, Dr Leslie Smith, and equipping an X-ray department – all on donations from those who believed in the demand for a hospital where women could rely on being treated by one of their own sex.

In contrast to today's practice, the medical staff were both

153

the initiators and final arbiters as regards hospital policy, but were handicapped in their ambitious desires by lack of endowment. There was always an endless chase to raise money. Mark Milbanke designed a special poster for the Appeal, Ruth Draper gave us a second matinee and Dame Madge Kendal was generosity itself over opening bazaars. Mrs Alec Holden was an indefatigable chairman of the Appeal Committee and one year she determined to stage a series of 'Living Pictures'. In my early days I was the only one of my family who could comfortably wear William Wilberforce's clothes. This was the more remarkable as he was a small man. Our shoulders and hips were apparently much the same size, but my legs were many inches longer so that the breeches were the only property that had to be specially made. Mrs Holden determined that one pair of pictures should be Hannah More with her dear friend William Wilberforce. So, carefully made up by the expert hand of E.R., I was duly framed and made to look, indeed I confess I felt like, my great grandfather; unexpectedly, I enjoyed the occasion. I had a momentary confidence that there was nothing I could not achieve while I wore his clothes!

It was an agreeable interlude in my medical work, for by this time I had been appointed a full Physician at the New Sussex and I had to go to London once weekly to see patients. I saw them at 39 Cadogan Gardens in the house of Mrs Rathbone, who had consulted me in Brighton. She had a retinal haemorrhage and was very deaf, but her courage and outlook on life taught me a great deal as to how to live undaunted with physical disabilities. She came to mean a great deal to me.

In May 1930 came the tragic shock of Lady Bell's death. Since the early Ibsen years she and E.R. had been the closest friends and corresponded regularly. Every literary project on either side was talked over and shared, as was every step regarding family and friends and travel. Several times a year E.R. would visit the Bells in Yorkshire. Political differences as to Women's Suffrage did not affect this devoted alliance and when they argued, some brilliant spark of humour from Lady Bell would bypass what seemed to be a head-on disagreement. Her death meant a gap which could never be filled.

In 1933 E.R. and Mrs Yates Thompson each gave me a Jersey cow from the Oving pedigree herd. Their names were Potentilla the fifth and Potpourri, and they were the foundation of my Jersey herd. We produced tuberculin tested clean milk and I learnt a great deal about human nature from my cows, as well as my landgirls. The bovine intelligence of Jerseys is certainly higher than Matriculation standard! Quite early in my cow keeping I agreed with my vet that one had to be versed in psychology to deal adequately with Jerseys.

[My Jerseys] were an everlasting solace amid the trials and problems of my practice. One of the greatest problems for any doctor is the chronic addiction to alcohol. One cold snow-bound winter's night early in my Brighton practice I was waked by a telephone call from a patient. The voice sounded desperate: 'Please, can you come round at once, it's my husband this time. It's most urgent.' I got there on my two feet as quickly as I could. I had not met Major X before. It was 3 a.m. and he was fully dressed in a tail coat, grey top hat, striped trousers and with a smart cane in his hand. He was a big, moustached, rather handsome man of about fifty years old and he was at the front door as I arrived.

'Get out of the way, I tell you. I shall be late as it is for Gatwick,' and he was roughly pushing aside his wife in dressing gown and a friend who were trying to bar the way.

'I'm Dr Wilberforce,' I said, and I shook his hand warmly and retained his clasp. 'It's cold in this passage. Come inside and talk to me first,' and I turned him round and propelled his staggering form into the bedroom. 'I'm fond of racing too, sometimes go to Goodwood – but this isn't the day for Gatwick.' We sat down together on the bed. He had waked from sleep, seen rats climbing the wall, become excited and finally, in spite of protests, dressed himself. Alcoholism was the diagnosis. I had not been long in practice but I had had plenty of hospital experience. With immense confidence I went on talking and finally convinced him that he wasn't well and he had made a mistake about Gatwick. He submitted to my undressing him, tucking him into bed and administering the necessary sedative. I then had to deal with his wife who was in tears and on the verge of a nervous breakdown. She was much amazed at her husband's docile submission to medical authority. Later that same day both husband and wife were once again rational people and, rather surprisingly, as long as they stayed in Brighton he kept sober. I think the rats had really frightened him.

[On the other hand] a patient may for a time be convinced that spirits taken in excess do have a cumulative poisoning effect on our internal organs, but this conviction unhappily becomes watered down sooner or later by temptation. Patients agree and promise all things, often most sincerely though unwillingly. One delightful lady tried very hard. Her illness, due to her habits, had frightened her; she was a competent business woman, a good companion with many top-grade financiers. She kept steady for quite a while, but there came a day when it had been very hot, and she rang and asked me to call. It was 'rather urgent'. I went, expecting to find her 'one over the eight', and telling myself that here was going to be another example of my failure to help. She greeted me warmly, had obviously not been at the bottle, said extravagant things about how much I'd helped her, how different she felt. Then most ingratiatingly: 'I want to make a proposal to you. You know some of my interests, and how easy it is for me to be in the know. I can give you a few tips on the Stock Exchange, and you can get in on the ground floor and increase your income substantially. Wouldn't you like that?' This conversation was at a moment when I was rather hard up and would have welcomed the prospect of more cash. I answered cautiously that I'd not much to invest anyhow, but – I paused and waited. 'All right then,' she said triumphantly, 'if you'll let me go back to gin again instead of white wine, particularly the morning gin, I'll give you two first-class tips.' My reactions were not slowed down by alcohol and I burst out laughing. She looked astonished and hurt; then I said seriously: 'You pay me to try and keep you well, and now you are proposing to bribe me to let you do what you know knocks you out. With your astute business brain, are you being logical do you think?' She wasn't happy, but she agreed and was quite friendly. Need I say she shortly afterwards changed her GP!

I learnt a lesson from a woman who came under my care a week after her husband had committed suicide. There was nothing much I could do for her and she had nothing to blame herself about; the poor man had had an incurable disease and he had chosen to take a short cut to the inevitable end. It was a fine summer and Sussex at its best, so I suggested one day that she might like to see the view from Chanctonbury Ring. We had climbed nearly to the top, making polite superficial talk, for I knew she was a reserved type whom I had no chance of approaching. Then she fell quite silent and dropped behind, and I walked slowly on for perhaps thirty or forty yards. When I looked back I saw her gazing over the weald with her back to me, lost to the world. I sat down and faced the summit of the hill with its beautiful Ring. I can't say how long it was before I heard her close behind me. 'Do forgive me, you must have thought me very rude. But I want you to know this walk has been a great help. More than you can imagine.' I said how glad I was that she had come. She went on and told me that since she was eighteen years old, when she had been very ill, she had never slept more than about four hours at night. Her parents and doctors were worried and tried all sorts of drugs but they only excited her. She grew to realise that she must accept this handicap. As time went on she had discovered for herself that she felt perfectly rested by the morning if she could collect, during the day, things of beauty; a picture, a person, a landscape, and study every line memorising them. At night she would lie and retrace every detail. She took away several views from Chanctonbury and she left me humble and grateful for the revelation of that mind. After that, when I came across patients who restlessly tossed till they impatiently turned to tranquillisers to dope them to sleep, I would try, by this story, to wean them from the habit. Their reaction was to assert they hadn't the time to waste over things like that. Occasionally, though, they would 'catch on' and then I would mentally wave a thankyou to Chanctonbury. How much it might be helpful in our hurried lives if we could set aside a little time to consider such examples of courage and beauty which are to be met with almost daily.

In 1937 I had under my care for a considerable period Aida Shaw, an overworked, broken-down little missionary, who was a cousin of Bernard Shaw's. She adored him, and his kindness to her was memorable. All I could do for her was to patch her up from time to time and keep her going, though I knew it was a losing battle. But she was a lion-hearted lady with a heavenly sense of humour and when we did strike a good patch, she was on top of the world. Early in February Aida Shaw was in the New Sussex and seriously ill, when one day the Matron rang me up to say she had two detectives in her office come to arrest Miss Shaw in connection with IRA activities. I dashed around and interviewed the police, vouched for her innocence (I was certain in my own mind this would not be her kind of frolic) and begged them to take no action for several days as she was desperately ill. They were rather concerned as to their duty but were completely understanding about it all. I immediately got in touch with George Bernard Shaw. Sir John Simon was Home Secretary and a friend of his, so G.B.S. wrote at once to beg him 'to take the Hove police off this mare's nest'. Swiftly came a long apologetic letter from Sir John Simon to George Bernard Shaw. The Hove police had been told to ferret out 'a Miss Shaw' and that was how the mistake had arisen.

Later on, when Aida was in extremis, I rang up George Bernard Shaw to warn him, but he wouldn't accept and face up to the fact that she was dying. He said: 'Oh no. Aida can't die. She won't.' The poor thing was unconscious, it was only a question of hours, and I was annoyed with George Bernard Shaw. All I could do was to obey the wishes she had expressed to me that, at her death, I should remove the suitcase she kept under her bed in the nursing home and get it back to him at Whitehall Court at once. It was crammed with letters from G.B.S. to his good little cousin.

Very rarely I considered whether this medical life was indeed the life of coveted independence I fought so hard to gain – a life of comparative slavery, it could be argued, to any Tom, Dick or Harry for twenty-four hours a day. And yet I maintain now, a life at least in my day, of the greatest happiness, however hurtful it might be to fight at times a losing battle against death; a life of great rewards, of incessant striving, of always being a learner at the foot of nature but, through it all, a life which gives a freedom, an independence of spirit, which can rarely be achieved in family and personal relationships.

12

VIRGINIA WOOLF'S LAST YEAR

1940–41

In 1939 we once again drifted into war. This time the Government, even if it had wished, had neither power nor occasion to limit the activities of women. They had, instead, plenty of opportunity to test their courage, endurance and adaptability.

It was in the early part of the war that I came to know Leonard and Virginia Woolf. They were living at Monks House, Rodmell, about ten miles from Brighton, and, for me, their friendship shone like a star in the sky over those dark days and nights of havoc and hard work. E.R.'s admiration for Virginia Woolf was boundless and she would talk endlessly of the power of her writing, her style, her sensitive dealing with character and the depth of her clear observations.

[E.R. had first met Virginia and Leonard Woolf in 1927] and was delighted when the Woolfs asked her to publish *Ibsen and the Actress* in the Hogarth Press Series the following year. Later, in 1935, Virginia Woolf had written to E.R. on behalf of Lydia Lopokova (Lady Maynard Keynes), asking her to come to a performance of *The Master Builder*, when Lydia Lopokova was to play Hilde. E.R. spent days worrying over how to answer this invitation for, though she would have done almost anything to please Virginia, she simply could not bring herself to watch another actress play this her best, her dearest part. Finally she went up to London and saw Virginia and told her exactly what she felt. She had been more apprehensive of this interview than I'd ever known her, but she returned greatly relieved and intensely appreciative of the sensitive way in which Virginia had at once accepted and understood her confession.

Virginia and Leonard came over to my house in Brighton

to have tea shortly before the publication in 1940 of [E.R.'s autobiography], *Both Sides of the Curtain*, which Virginia had been given to read in proof. E.R. wanted to discuss possible titles, and they had a long tete-a-tete before coming to a decision. When we had seen the Woolfs into their car and they had driven away, E.R. seized me by the arm and, with shining eyes, burst out, 'Do you know what Virginia said to me? "Your mind interests me so much!"' And she added in awe-struck tones, '*This* from Virginia Woolf!'

That was the first time I had seen Virginia Woolf. I was concerned about her extreme thinness and was delighted when she tucked into our home-made bread and kind Mrs Yates Thompson's butter. We went over to Monks House on one or two occasions after that, and in May 1940 we attended a lecture Virginia gave in Brighton on *The Leaning Tower*, when my clinical eye was again troubled by her thinness.

All this time [E.R.'s brother] Raymond was cabling more and more urgently for E.R. to return to America. She was very reluctant to leave England for her whole heart was devoted to this country and had been since she came in 1888, though she was quite determined not to be naturalised and had never agreed with Henry James about his gesture of allegiance to Britain in the 1914 war. Lady Buxton, too, begged her to return to the safety of America and to get away from the police restrictions – as an alien she had to register whenever she moved – and the difficulties over food. Finally, after the last American ship had sailed and under pressure of yet more cables from Raymond, she submitted and we set about planning her departure.

This was a formidable task as there was no ship available and the only possible chance was somehow to manoeuvre a flight to Lisbon and thence on by clipper. Every source was tapped and finally a seat was promised to Lisbon, while Raymond in America was pulling every string to get a seat in a clipper. But there was still an apparently insurmountable obstacle, for she stoutly refused to leave England unless she might take her notes of the unfinished earlier chapters of Volume Two of her autobiography. There was a regulation that no printed matter or manuscript should leave the country, not even a manuscript dealing only with the 1890s. Finally I went to see Dr Thomas Jones, who had been Deputy Secretary to the Cabinet. He was a friend of Mrs Yates Thompson's, and both E.R. and I knew him and appreciated his kindly, humorous way of dealing with difficult problems. He had not served under five Prime Ministers without learning more than a little about the art of getting things done. No one could have been more ready to help, but he stressed the difficulties. Of course it was nonsense, he agreed, and there was no likelihood of there being information in such a packet which might help the enemy. But I realised, didn't I, that the Government could take no risks? I pleaded the case with intense urgent appeal. Finally he said he would think about what could be done. At last we heard from 'T.J.' If I took along the packet, he said, he would personally seal it with a written guarantee that he had inspected the contents and vouched for there being nothing which could imperil this country if it fell into enemy hands. With his reputation this would ensure the safe transit of the precious packet. I remember now the appearance of that large stout envelope, sealed back and front, and in all corners with Dr Thomas Jones's large and impressive seal.

1940 was a piping hot summer, and E.R., who always hated the heat, was completely spent by her preparations and the packing of trunks which were to be sent on by sea. It was with a saddened, anxious heart that I watched the small aeroplane take to the air. When she arrived in Lisbon the heat was oppressive. The town was crammed to overflowing with refugees fleeing from Europe and, after one or two uncomfortable nights in a stuffy hotel bedroom, the doctor, who had been summoned, moved E.R. to the British Hospital. Ill and miserable though she might be, E.R.'s courage never failed her when travelling, particularly when she had an enthralling book to sustain her. She wrote from her hospital bed [about Virginia Woolf's latest book, a biography of Roger Fry, written most reluctantly in response to urgent appeals from Fry's sister and his mistress]:

In the day and in the night I have read Virginia. A queer

book – product of a loyalty and a self-suppression rarely equalled I should think. V. is immensely handicapped by the fact of Fry's living relatives and what they would expect. No wonder she called the thing 'a difficult biography'. The life of such a genius [Roger Fry] was worth writing, whether at Virginia's expenditure, who am I to say. She couldn't escape doing a remarkable thing. She saved me many a trying moment in my own latest Queer Pilgrimage by giving me the refuge of her pages and the support of her crystal mind.

E.R. hated her exile (the United States had not yet joined the Allies) and I tried to keep her in the picture as to my activities. She was feeling very cut off and far away from what was happening in England. [I also] encouraged her to get on with Volume Two, the planned sequel to her autobiography, *Both Sides of the Curtain*. I told her such incidents of the war in Brighton as I thought the Censor would pass, but I knew that what would most interest her would be a record of my visits to the Woolfs at Rodmell. I asked Virginia to write a word of encouragement to E.R., as I knew this would be an enormous stimulus to her:

> Monks House,
> Rodmell, Lewes, Sussex.

17 November 1940

Dear Miss Robins,

I heard from Octavia the other day that you have reached America safely. Now I calculate you must have had your three weeks to recover. So, am I being impertinent and intrusive if I write to ask – are you going on with your book? I know from experience that either one is going on, or has good reasons for not going on. All the same I can't help putting to you the reader's case; which is simply, please if you can, give us another volume. Most books come to an end and one forgets them. But your book hasn't come to an end, and I haven't forgotten it. Thus you have put me into the position of a spider, dangling at the end of a thread, which it can't attach to anything, unless you will help it. I implore you to have pity on Virginia suspended on a thread. And I believe you have left lots of people in the same predicament. Well, I won't say any more except that I beg of you to go on. And if this comes at the wrong moment, please forgive me.

This moment, here in my garden room, happens to be so lovely I can't keep my eyes on the paper. A bomb burst the river bank and we are flooded all over the marsh. The sea comes almost to our gate. And the gardener has just called me to come and look at a swan. So you see the bombs so far have been kind to us. I suspect we seem, at a distance, far worse than we seem to ourselves. I hope to see Octavia some day. And end with our affectionate double regards – Leonard's and mine.

> Yours,
> Virginia Woolf

I then suggested that, as milk was rationed and food was difficult, I might send the Woolfs my Jersey milk and cream regularly and so help them to withstand the influenzal infection which was prevalent just then. Virginia agreed to this by letter:
'Oh yes we will eat your cream gratefully and defy the flu – *But* we have loads of apples. Also books. So let's make a barter.'
I wrote to E.R. in December 1940:

I went to tea with the Woolfs and I found them apologising for untidiness (books and wine bottles and cases in process of being unpacked as the result of their having to salvage some of what was left of their London quarters) and most friendly. She told me she had written to you, but was scared lest her saying anything to you about your writing should enrage (that was her term), as 'authors are very queer people'. I assured her that I knew there was no one who would have so much influence upon you as she. This she did not accept. In subsequent talk, she said that she hated to be written to about her work, as people often annoyed her, by for instance saying, 'When are you going to give us more criticism?', which to her sensitiveness meant they did not want any more novels.

They said, of course, how much they liked you and recalled when they had first met you; she as a child when you were acting Ibsen, I gather. [Virginia described her first conversation with E.R. in 1927] 'When Miss Robins came up and said such sensitive, understanding things to me, and I think mentioned my mother, I longed to talk to her, and I was immediately impressed by her personality and quite overwhelmed.' She had been much impressed by your modesty, had thought it so extraordinary that you should have valued so much her view of Volume one, as she felt that you were so great that her view should not have mattered to you. I recalled how you looked upon Virginia as probably the greatest living writer of English prose. This she showed disbelief at, but did, I think, finally accept simply and rather touchingly. She said that she had never read any of your novels and she could not think why, and she specially wanted to read *The Open Question*, which Hugh Walpole had said was even better than *The Magnetic North*. Anyhow when I got home I very nobly sent her my only copy of *The Open Question*, since you pinched my little red one.

Leonard asked whether you ever really relaxed; you were always so perfect when they'd seen you he couldn't imagine your doing so. Virginia went through your *Both Sides of the Curtain* and the parts she had been impressed by. How fascinating you must have been that all these people, the best of the 1890s, should have gone out of their way to help you. Why didn't you, since you were so successful, stay on the stage? Interesting your meeting Oscar [Wilde], and others. 'But of course,' says Leonard, 'it is in a sense all preparatory to the most interesting time she must have had over Ibsen,' and his eyes shone. I liked them so much in their appreciation of you. They were so simple and unaffected about it all. There's no doubt she regards you with no little awe. Thought so enthralling the fact that it was so intimately about the Theatre, 'I know nothing, and have always wanted to know about the stage, so was thrilled by it,' she said.

I also said that as a doctor I felt that prevention was much the most important side of Medicine, and that if I might be allowed to send her some more Devonshire cream as a small return for the pleasure she had given me by her books, I would feel myself privileged.

On 23 December 1940, I wrote to E.R.:

I went over with Devonshire cream to the Woolfs. I thought having done my duty all around I'd give myself a treat. Moreover, if Hitler is going to invade or be nasty I'd a feeling I'd get all I could done before Christmas Eve. I marched up the path and greet Leonard and dog and he takes basket with cream and says he'll fill it with apples in return for cream. A barter scheme which entirely suits me. Find Virginia inside with hands worse than icicles. I say how truly grateful I am to her and report your cable saying 'Virginia's letter sets me to work again.' She turns her back on me rather shyly and hearing the end turns round with a beaming and delightful smile, 'Say it again!' I obey. And to hide her extreme pleasure she makes for kitchen to get the teapot.

She had been sorting papers, love letters from her father to her mother. Had been swept away by them. 'Poor Leonard is tired out by my interest in my family and all it brings back.' I say how I'd stayed with Mrs Yates Thompson and how much I'd gathered they liked Leslie Stephen [Virginia's father].

I wrote to Virginia about the milk question and had a letter back, on a quite clean sheet of paper, headed:

This sheet of paper came out of our bombed house – that's the dirt on it – bombs.

Monks House,
Rodmell.
31 December.
Dear Octavia,
I never heard a more absurd 'business proposition' as you

call it. A month's milk and cream in return for an unborn and, as far as I can tell, completely worthless book. I've lost all power over words – can't do a thing with them. What we suggest is that if you would send your bounty, say Monday and Friday, to Lewes we would meet it. And return – well, apples? That's about the only thing we can return. Milk and cream are at the moment worth tons of apples. We know this, and can only put it on record that we realise it all – your generosity, and the trouble, and the really miraculous gift.

Your quotations, far from enraging, put me up a peg. Of course the Roger Fry was more or less an experiment in self suppression, as E.R. guessed. But I was afraid I'd somehow suppressed him too. It was a touch and go business – either too much colour or too little. But on the whole, I'd rather there were no biographer, than a mix up of the two. I suppose the really expert somehow combine both, rightly.

You can't write long enough letters to *this* author – but, having been book lugging, up at our hired room, I can't, as you see, make my hand cease to tremble. Now as a doctor, your hand is firm. So you can write. One of Roger's eccentricities was that he never analysed character, but always art – I daresay the reasons for his mastery. Let me know about the bargain.

I wrote to E.R.:

I like to see the Woolfs and be intellectually roused by them. I rang up Leonard to ask would they like some cream and may I bring it over after Out Patients? I've had a thumping success in taking Devonshire cream made by Maud to Leonard and Virginia. And I'm so glad. They both look thin and half-starved and if ever anybody ought to benefit from my herd it should be those waifs. Waifs I'm sure they are about food. Anyhow, I've arranged to barter my dairy produce in exchange for apples and, say I cheerfully, a copy of Virginia's next book. At the moment she says she has no power over words and can't write. (N.B. I think our dear friend loves to exaggerate. All Clear gone, that's nice and early.) And then, 'What shall I do? A novel, another biography, criticism?'

O.W., 'Well, you don't expect me to say, as you have lots in your head. And in any case . . .' I was going on to say she had herself told me that she was enraged by people wanting this or that and inferring they didn't like t'other, when she chipped in, 'Yes, I've lots of ideas germinating, but I want to know what the public wants. You're one of my public.' I, of course, with complete inadequacy, plus native caution, said nothing!

In a letter to Virginia Woolf on 3 January 1941, asking them to lunch before a concert and arguing about the barter for milk, I wrote:

If you try to weigh things on a balance it would take a sea of milk before I got even with you. My greatest joy in life has always been reading and you have given me untold delight and helped me at many a difficult moment. You have stimulated and helped E.R. as no one else can or could. And, moreover, please let me have a hand in being constructive. You see my job is nearly all either patching or regretting that God hadn't asked my advice! Much of practice is therefore spent in being humiliated by one's limitations. Now, to cherish an illusion that with enough extra milk you might both go ahead and write your greatest masterpieces is a great and cheering thought. I'm so glad you feel you've 'lost all power over words'. Go on and abandon yourself to that feeling; every true genius has to lie fallow for a time while the seed germinates – as you know perfectly well. So I'm quite unmoved; instead merely reassured as to the certainty about my part of the bargain.

As to Roger Fry, I can imagine no more really expert biographer. Have you been thinking of writing your father's life? I expect that's cheek and I grovel in advance! You said authors are touchy and I'm suddenly brought up against that warning and am not sure where I've got to, as I really know you very little. Or is it that the remote cousinship makes an illusion that I feel I know you . . . well, *better* than I know my near cousins?

This allusion was due to the fact that William Wilberforce's sister married the first James Stephen – an ardent abolitionist, an ancestor to Virginia. I go on to offer to lug books to save her strength. On 9 January 1941 I had another letter from Virginia:

Oh dear – now you've telephoned, and I was just about to write. We can't come to the concert, as Leonard lectures and there's the Blackout and the Chairs to see to. I'm sorry. Think of eating Turkey! and I want to continue the argument – the very one-sided argument: books versus cream. I don't see how you can brave it out. Nothing we both ever to the end write can outweigh your milk and cream at this bitter and barren moment.

This hand doesn't shake from book lugging, but from rage. Louie being gone to a funeral, I cooked lunch: and the rice floored me. That's why I rage. I am now consulting a cookery book. So how am I to write *your* book? My father's been done already – F.W. Maitland. But I'm too rice-infested to make any sense, so forgive; and I'm sorry I forgot to answer before.

On 15 January I wrote to E.R.:

I have hoped that my visits to the Woolfs would stimulate and stir you. Do they? I can't quite be sure of my own diagnosis yet. But I'm pretty sure of certain things – that physically they're both frail. But to go on about Virginia. At first I felt she'd exaggerate to make any sort of amusing story – but about her craft, your writing, any good writing and her own efforts, I don't feel she's the same person. That's the side I like and admire – the respect for words, the constructive artist, the builder and architect passionately concerned that each brick is well and truly laid – nay, is perfectly placed in the one and only perfect position. That's the Virginia that makes me feel I'm a nitwit and makes one want to start afresh and stretch one's brain.

I had entertained Virginia with the description of our fire watching in the Montpelier Crescent Area. We had a meeting at my house and formed a committee. At one moment it was said that women should only watch for incendiaries through the windows and they should of course go home to bed at midnight. The chairman was most emphatic over this; he didn't think it right for the ladies of the neighbourhood to be out after midnight, and he knew that the married men of his audience would stoutly support this suggestion. At this last remark I suddenly lost my temper, and got up and said that as a doctor I wished strongly to protest; at this stage of the world's history we were all in equal danger, and that there should be any sort of sex distinction seemed to me utter nonsense. The chairman gasped with amazement, and all the elderly ladies and a few men warmly clapped this remark.

I had been away from Brighton on the saddest visit I had yet experienced, and profoundly unhappy, I wrote to Virginia on 26 January:

Dear Virginia,

You were uncommon kind to tell me about your new venture the last time I saw you and I'd promised myself the joy of writing to you, after I'd had time to think about it, last Sunday. But instead I was sent for on that Saturday by my old beloved friend, Mrs Yates Thompson, because, as I now realise, she felt she was dying.

It was as poignant and searing a few days as I can remember, only made bearable by the fact that she had surprisingly summoned me. She had that gay, gallant courage such as I've come to feel one rarely meets except in the Victorians, and she kept it to the finish. First rate brains, admirable judgement – a complete despot, household and relations scared of her. Yet she was a very shy person, a well of reserve and discretion. In these days one ought not to grieve when an old lady dies as she would have wished, I believe (I mean no long illness, etc.). But I don't like to feel one of one's foundations demolished. Before I'd even got as far as the School of Medicine, she quite irrationally encouraged me to think I'd be useful in Medicine. And without her I don't believe I could have started here in practice seventeen years ago. She breeds pedigree Jerseys and gave me my first cow, Pot Pourri, seven years ago – so it's to her we owe the cream.

About your new book, I'm inclined to think it's just what is most needed now, and after the war. I come across a lot of people who are starving for good books. One friend (Dr John Ryle), consulting physician, was poignant a few months ago about the need for good stuff over the radio – as he said, the Spaniards had been so helped and heartened by good prose and poetry. (He has been meeting the Blitz at Guys Hospital – living there. And has a more than average brain.) But for the ordinary, haphazard public, we all want a common guide. With your 'crystal clear' intelligence, for which one thanks the Gods continually, you can distil out the essence in comparatively small space. I feel that unless we all get back to some sort of settled good reading, we'll lose our sense of proportion and thought (if any). It will mean we'll be so standardised in our minds by newspapers and wireless, as most of the world is, in its uniformed clothes now. And Hitler and co. have played on just that note – it's a great simplification of life to be told what to wear, do, think, even eat! And it appeals to the lazy side of man, so that existence becomes almost as low a job as any other form of animal life.

Monday. I can tell you this, reaching for something to bite into, I came to the conclusion the other day, after tackling bits of four very different authors, none modern, that it is just amazing how gently and effortlessly and completely you hold one's mind. On this occasion it was – is – *Night and Day* that does the trick. Wasn't it A.E. Housman who rather belittled the sense in poetry and said it was the jingle, the arrangement, of the words that really mattered? You not only have the brilliantly clarifying effect for the mind, but you also arrange the jingle so that it soothes the ear, which isn't a bit fair on other writers.

And now your kind letter has come. I'm relieved to know you can still eat. I'm quite unperturbed that you say you can't write. The longer you feel like that the better you'll write when you do get really going. So just don't try. Pot Pourri and her descendants are standing up to all claims with complete confidence, so there's plenty of cream to come. Don't get tired and keep Louie 'to it'. I'll ring up probably one day early next week and suggest coming over. I look forward enormously to that, and it's angelic of you to have me.

> Love and blessings,
> Your
> O.W.

On 31 January 1941 I wrote to E.R.:

I went over to W's [the Woolfs] today. Took them some calycanthus since Leonard is such a great gardener. He was thrilled by it – so was she, only she's a vaguer, less expressive person. Those two citizens are nice folk. She looks thinner and thinner, says she's teaching herself to cook in order to be ready for anything. 'After the war we certainly shan't get anybody to do for us – and at any moment we may have to do for ourselves' – this not on financial but general grounds. And I gave her various recipes.

And I suddenly felt how deep and solid her affection is for him – how real and rooted. There's no doubt they're both a highly sensitive couple. And she takes life hard. I've a suspicion that they both quite like to see me for my comparative stolidity. She also told me a little of her, mainly past, worries. Headaches, etc. And I gather, even now, she can't work long at a stretch, never after tea – and often breaks off when rather desperate, and goes and makes a pudding or something. If you ask me, I think she is a thoroughly frail creature and I wish we could do something to binge her up.

I told her on Friday that I was very unobservant and didn't notice environments often – or what people wore, or even if they were or were not good looking. She looked a little surprised and then said: 'No, but you look for their character.' I *didn't* say I, as a reflex, absorbed their physical fitness and disabilities to a large extent.

On 23 February Virginia wrote:

You've reduced me not to silence quite, but to a kind of splutter – I mean, the cream, the cheese, the milk. And I don't see how to begin: and twice this week the debt mounts. And you don't come here so that I could speak by word of mouth. Dear, dear – I'm dumb. But can just say we had a magnificent feast of cheese last night: not had one since September and seldom any so suave and sweet and yet sour. No I didn't add sugar. For there was a natural sweetsour in it that was best unmixed.

We too have been turmoiled, not, I expect, for any such good purpose as you. Only going to Cambridge, to Letchworth, and somehow having a run of visitors in the house. Should you be able to come over, please suggest it.

On 28 February I wrote to E.R.:

Today I went over to Virginia and Leonard's. They'd had visitors. Quentin [Bell], the nephew, had devoured all Leonard's marmalade! Also Vita [Sackville West]. Not, I gather, at the same moment. She had brought them butter. But I can't say I think *my* milk ministrations are doing much good. She, Virginia, looks a better colour but is still as thin as a razor.

I honestly think they like to see me. They most affectionately ask after you. Full of a kind solicitude. We'd a long discussion on *Three Guineas*. She said that work had brought more letters and fury than any book she'd ever written. Did *I* think it overstated and shrill? Indeed no. V.W. been asked to be the one woman on the London Library and she was writing to refuse. She doesn't hold with all these honorary degrees or titles. So she's always trying to tell her young woman friends that they are merely sops, and until thrown open entirely equally not to be accepted. Do you agree? (*Yes. Yes.* Written in by E.R.!)

Then, 'Can you help me make up my mind?' Her brother-in-law, Clive [Bell], had rung up to say that the Hamish Hamiltons wanted her to go to lunch on Sunday. Had saved up some, but not all, petrol. Would therefore call at Lewes on Sunday to pick up Virginia and Clive and take 'em to Blackboys (miles away East) and bring 'em back to Lewes. Thence by bus. Would mean starting at 11.30 and interrupting her work. And she couldn't make up her mind. 'Leonard doesn't want me to go as he thinks it means such a big slice of the day, and not interesting enough. But I think they might be stimulating, and I'm susceptible and they might give me champagne, mentally as well.' Leonard interrupted, 'Yes, but you'd be in their power and Clive, once he got talking, might go on for hours and you'd not be able to break away and get back.' I finally decided that she'd better not go and she pretended that she'd take my advice. I wonder. [Virginia did not go, 'and got into hot water with her brother-in-law for not doing so.' Octavia was 'glad about that'.]

We also went more into her book, having your letter in which you aren't keen, and I boldly asked about her proportions. Not a *history* [of literature] at all – merely criticism, rather like the *Common Reader*, only giving hints as to the development of writing. Quite short, I gathered, and more or less to please Duncan Grant. I said I thought you'd approve more of that – as I knew you loved the Common Readers. Leonard keen on the sort of criticism that Matthew Arnold had done.

Then, as I got up to go, she looks at me gravely in that detached way, and says: 'I think I'd like to do a sketch of you, would you mind?' She'd been talking about Roger Fry just before, and for a moment I took this literally (i.e. paints!) 'Yes, I've already a picture of you as a child at Lavington, beautiful name, and you could talk to me. You see, I think it would be rather fun to do portraits of living people – anonymously of course.' I say, hunting round in my embarrassment, and not being sure whether to be flattered or annoyed, and feeling frankly bewildered, I say, 'But if it were good – er – it would be recognised and then – er – in my profession I should be had up for advertising,' and I appeal to Leonard. He non-committal, but considers in his judicial way there might be something in that. She then says: 'Oh, then you wouldn't like it.' At which I think of you and how *you'd* perhaps like it and say: 'Oh, I think I'm really immensely flattered and I think it might be rather . . . fun,' lamely. 'Well, I might try and send it you to see what you think?' And I made off, feeling I'd better hurriedly escape – and longing for your guidance in the matter.

On 4 March I had a letter from Virginia:

And now of course typing don't suit any other [personal] kind of letter. So I won't begin on the question of my living portrait. All I say is, I see that no one can be asked to sit. Why should they? Wouldn't it be a kind of torture? It was only a wild flitting dream. All the same, I add in handwriting, I think you're very paintable, as the painters say. Now I wonder why? Something that composes well. Perhaps reticence and power combined: – then there's the garden at Lavington.

I will try to write to Miss Robins. No, no, no, I cannot write on a typewriter, and so must give over and say once more, what a damned generous woman you are. Have you any use for bottled gooseberries? Many pots here if you would take them.

On 13 March Virginia had written to E.R.:

I was very sorry to hear from Octavia that you had had an accident. Selfishly, I'm afraid it may interfere with the book that I'm looking forward to. But I remember a saying of Henry James – all experiences are of use to a writer. I think he was talking about a nervous breakdown. So may it be with a broken bone.

I now go on to say that I've been cycling into Lewes – not a very interesting remark, save that it connects with Octavia. Has she told you, I wonder – no, I don't suppose she has – of her amazing bi-weekly bounty – cream, milk, sometimes a cheese? That's what I've been fetching. You can't think how it brightens our weekly bill of fare. Also, to fetch her empty basket, she sometimes comes over, and this has been, is, and will be, I hope, a great treat. Is it our drop of blood in common? Anyhow we sit over the fire, as if we'd known each other in the woods at Lavington. It's odd how our lives have run, just not meeting, but through the same country. That's the sort of woman I most admire – the reticence, the quiet, the power. Here I can imagine her look of enquiry – why? Well, it's difficult to say why. It's the variety and the calm partly. As you can imagine, she's healing the sick by day, and controlling the fires by night.

At this moment there's a flood of yellow flowers in the garden – and the view from my window is like a block of flawed emerald, half green, half blue. It's amazingly peaceful here – you can almost hear the grass grow; and the rooks are building. You wouldn't think that at 7.30 the planes will be over. Two nights ago they dropped incendiaries, in a row, like street lamps, all along the downs. Two haystacks caught and made a lovely illumination – but no flesh was hurt. Indeed, every bomb they drop only casts up a crater so far. It's difficult I find to write. No audience. No private stimulus, only this outer war. And in these circumstances, Octavia is very refreshing. Leonard asks me to add his respects to my love, and we both often think of you and the book.

In another letter to E.R. on 14 March, I say:

And you approve of Virginia's idea? Bless me. I nearly turned it down. That was my first instinct. Then I began to feel a bit flattered that *her* mind should want to tackle me as a subject. Then I thought how you'd be pleased. Then she wrote the letter I sent you. To which I replied, 'Should I come over on Wednesday and collect two pots of gooseberries (barter for milk)'; and as to 'torture to sit' – I had an unanalytical mind and it would be marvellous to talk to a born clarifier. She rang up and I went over, after nearly a whole night out firewatching and a heavy Out Patient's. Found them having tea. (Nearly ran away on the doorstep, with sudden stage fright!) After tea, upstairs to little room where you sat and Leonard and Virginia talked. Presently Leonard says he'd better leave us to it. Virginia says something to hold him and he stays another ten minutes. (They *do* work well together.) Then he picks up some proofs, says he must get back to his work, and will leave us to our 'seance' and goes off. Virginia moves to his chair on side of fireplace and says tactfully (wily V!) she had been feeling desperate – depressed to the lowest depths, had just finished a story. Always felt like this – but specially useless just now. The Village wouldn't even allow her to firewatch – could do nothing – whereas *my* life . . . *No*, I say firmly, and point out that only she could write as she does and so on.

'Leonard says I shouldn't think about myself so much and I should think more about outside things.' I say how my job does too much of that, lames one too much and knocks out concentration.

'No, not when you're actually on a case.' How did *she* know?

'No,' I agree 'not at the actual moment. But afterwards, reading, writing, anything, it's all interruption.'

'Yes, but people *need* you. You're doing something worthwhile, practical.' I agree that, except at times immediately after a book is out and reviews are tumbling over themselves, a writer hasn't the advantage of the stage, where the audience pulls the best out of him. And then suddenly we talk of Lavington and my childhood. I can't remember when it was – ages ago – but I must have said something of Lavington garden, as she says she sees the background and the beauty and peace.

'But had you no dark and depressing times?' Poor Virginia – thirteen when her mother died – her [half-sister, Stella] died at twenty-five and both were irreparable blows. And her father rather went to pieces, I think, after her mother's death and 'threw himself too much upon us. Made too great emotional claims upon us and that I think has accounted for many of the wrong things in my life. I never remember any enjoyment of my body.' I questioned what she meant. 'You adored the woods and games – I never had that chance.' It was all for her, I gather, intellectual and emotional – no healthy outdoor outlet.

And as we talked one thing became clear to me. Her interest in me, I believe, is because I'm the farthest possible opposite to her own build-up. Outside interests, physical toughness and game loving, as against that narrowed introspective, searching, restless, rather hauntingly fearful but brilliant mind. She said she envied me my touch with reality. Did I never make notes of any of the interesting things that came my way. And, next minute, 'drink in women. Was it curable?' She had a friend – gifted poetically – and a little more description, and I thought I knew whom she meant. You can guess, I'm sure. Very distressed about this.

Heaven knows what impression she got at the end of an hour. But I know I interested and surprised and took her out of herself. And isn't that an achievement in these grim days, for that rather unhappy, haunted-by-the-past, gifted genius? And I got a pretty shrewd picture of her in the process.

Oh! and I told her at the start, that the basis of medicine, science, was to try to be truthful – whereas for her, I inferred, that it wasn't so important. But my immediate difficulty was to be sure of what was the truth. I might have added that I spent my time living ahead and not in the past. Again the reverse of that backward-looking spirit.

Sunday 16th. I've no idea of the dimensions or anything else she wants to do this job – nor I think has she entirely. What worries me a bit is how far she'll use anything that, as regards my family, might hurt feelings. But does this really matter? I gather she had attempted somebody else and not been pleased with it. I didn't ask who it was though I wouldn't mind asking her about anything; she and Leonard are the frankest couple I've met on short acquaintance. But I feel she's the most highly sensitive, easily hurt person and I'd handle her as gently as I could. During part of the last war was when she lost hold and I've a feeling back of my head that she's a bit scared this may happen again. In which case, anybody as bucolic and hefty and – what am I? *tranquillising* perhaps – may help her somewhat.

Have you finished *Night and Day*? Please do. I'm sure Katherine is greatly like her in many ways.

After Mrs Yates Thompson's death it was suggested that E.R. should write a Portrait of this remarkable, modest, reserved woman. Mrs Reginald Smith and the Woolfs were eager that the project should be accomplished as quickly as possible, and it was my task to supply accurate data, [as I informed E.R.:]

Saturday 22 March 1941

Yesterday I went over to the Woolfs again. They are most interested in Mrs Yates Thompson's Portrait. 'What an interesting character and I specially like the latter half,' says Leonard. Virginia was intrigued over our beloved friend's general make-up. Virginia by way of being down but looking rather better colour than often. Wanted to know more of my youth. What my first impressions of you were. For my part, what I seem to gain is, by bits and pieces, a picture of Virginia's earlier years or anyhow what she was like. She asked me yesterday if I'd ever read *Orlando*.

'Oh yes,' I said brightly.

'What did you think of it?'

'Immensely clever as far as I remember.'

'Well that was a fantastic biography and *Roger Fry* is the other I've attempted and both are failures. And I don't know exactly how I'd do you; probably more like Orlando – but I can't write. I've lost the art. But you are doing more useful work, helping things on.' So then I tell her how far more important her work is and try to buck her up. 'Yes, but I'm buried down here – I've not the stimulation of seeing people. I can't settle to it.' I say she's making this an excuse, making the war an excuse. And it's a difficult time to concentrate now. But she's got to do it and stick to it. Golly, what I wouldn't give to be able to write as she can.

I said I thought this family business was all nonsense, blood thicker than water – balderdash. Surprised her anyway. I'm sure *she* thinks far too much of it! She said she had taken to scrubbing floors when she couldn't write – it 'took her mind off'. She's too taken up with her own mind and its reactions. It would do *her* the world of good to harrow a field or play a game.

I finish my letter with comments on Mrs Yates Thompson. The Portrait was shortly to be printed privately by the Hogarth Press.

I had succumbed to influenza after my visit to Monks House and on 26 March I wrote to E.R.:

I'm lying in bed at 11 a.m. (first day of temperature down) when telephone bell rings. *Leonard*. Wants my professional help. About her. And then he pours out his difficulties and fears, and *her* fears. She had said she wouldn't see me but, he sounded desperate, things were getting too bad and he felt he must have help. I'm in a cleft stick. *Can* I help. Can I get to her as regards my own legs? But one knows what the stimulation of an urgent appeal is and I conceal my bedbound state and finally arrange that he brings her here at 3.15 unless she jibs. I feel that I can do more to impress her professionally in my own surroundings; easier to get across when I'm in charge of the environment. So, later, he rang up to confirm appointment.

And they came. Oh, but it was rocky going. I forgot to cough and entirely lost my own sensations of weakness in a battle of – not wits, but *minds*.

'*Quite* unnecessary to have come.' Wouldn't answer my questions frankly (though I asked rather few, for me) and was generally resistive. I met each phase patiently.

'All you have to do is to reassure Leonard.' Finally, after I gently and firmly told her that I knew her answer wasn't true and that she really felt . . . I outlined this. She began in her sleep-walking way at my request to get undressed. Stopped.

'Will you promise if I do this not to order me a rest cure?' *Blast*, say I to myself. I look her confidently in the eye: 'What I promise you is that I won't order you anything you won't think it reasonable to do. Is that fair?' She agreed. And we went on with the exam. – she protesting at each stage like a petulant child!

Well, at the end we start off again and talk. And then she does confess her fears. That the past will recur – that she won't be able to work again and so on. Tragic. God knows if I did her a penn'orth of good. But I had some inspirations. '*Because* you'd had trouble and come through it – shouldn't this be a reassurance to you that if you'll take things easy now . . . If you have an appendix operation it leaves a scar on your body but that's all and you forget about it – if you have a mental illness it leaves a scar on your memory perhaps but that's all. It's only if you think about these things that it matters.' Oh, I expect I did no real good. But I threw in somewhere, putting out my hand and clasping her icy cold one, 'If you'll collaborate I know I can help you, and there's nobody in England I'd like more to help.' She looked a little less strained and perhaps a trifle detachedly pleased! But the *poignancy* of it all. And *can* I help?

At the one moment I'd almost a thought of Backset for her, but the risk is great I feel. However, if ever we took any risk it must be with her, I feel you'd say, as regards Backset's good name, eh? Anyhow, I'm very busy at the minute and she's the sort of case that needs time. Oh dear! Well, I'm going back to bed soon to get rid of the aches and gird myself anew for the next trial.

In the midst of my talk after with Leonard, machine gunning followed by a crump. I hope something brought down. But we neither felt it of interest or importance by comparison with the matter in hand. I continued to drive home my points. 'No writing or criticism for a month. She has been too much nurtured on books. She never gets away from them. Let her be rationed and then she'll come good again. *If* she'll collaborate.'

March 27 1941

Was it only last night I wrote to you? I'm still pretty weak after the 'flu and only saw Davy of all my patients today. But early I wrote and sent by the milk what I hoped might be a reassuring, gentle, friendly note to Virginia (who could not have got it). Just after lunch about two I rang up. No reply. Troubled, a little haunted by a look I surprised yesterday, I rang again at 6.30. Leonard answers: 'A dreadful catastrophe has happened.' Poor distraught unhappy people. She slipped off about twelve – leaving a note behind – they dragged the river, he had found her stick at the edge. I'm greatly shocked and most unhappy. Rang up Ryle [Dr John Ryle, consulting physician and friend of O.W.]; told him all I'd discovered yesterday. He, bless him, comforting, reassuring. Said at once same condition as Pam's (I'd felt this but had sheered off it) and that if it hadn't been today it would inevitably have been sooner or later, whatever any of us had done; and that if I'd taken drastic steps yesterday and suggested a nursing home, it would only have precipitated it last night. And I did right in giving her a chance. Isn't it all tragic?

I so much wish now that I had gone over more often and tried to get hold of her more as a friend. But, as you know, I'm shy and I always felt her aloofness and I had a horror of possibly boring that highly intellectual, cultivated mind, so I consciously rationed myself of visits. Though I believe they always did like me to go. And since she had this portrait idea it gave me an excuse – but no, it would not have helped. She was desperate and scared, and, my belief is, haunted by her father. I said this to Leonard and he agreed. 'We've been so happy together,' she said to me yesterday of their marriage. She also felt acutely not being able to do anything about the war. And I had thought I was clever in quoting what she herself had said about Jane Austen and the Napoleonic Wars and getting on with her job all the time. She had smiled quite naturally and been pleased about my throwing back her own words at her. Oh *damn*. I did so hope I could help.

It is hateful to be so powerless in my job – Mrs Yates Thompson and now Virginia. Oh dear – head is bloody all right but it takes a bit of doing to keep it unbowed sometimes.

March 28

To continue. Still no news. They are still dragging the river and until they are successful there can be no inquest I believe. I talk to Leonard on 'phone. Finally, after lunch am so *haunted* by Virginia and my own failure to help and thinking round in circles that I feel, 'If I'm like this what is Leonard going through?' So I ring up; would he like me to go over for a short while? Very much, says he. I go and we discuss her whole life medically and what specialists she had seen, etc. How, when Leonard married her, he knew nothing of her affliction. Its recurring nature – the many advices. Her happy nature. His completely truthful direct way of dealing with her condition to her. Finally I think we agreed that it was the association of the 1914 War and her worst phase that had haunted her mind now and convinced her a similar happening in this war was likely. He asked if, when I talked to her, I felt she was paying attention. I said frankly that I'd gathered from what she said from time to time that she was depressed and needing distraction – and I had had an odd feeling that I did distract and bring her a certain amount of peace. He looked relieved and said he had hoped that might be so.

When I came away, picking my way down the narrow stairs, I say over my shoulder, 'As a doctor one thing strikes me very forcibly, that you were Heaven inspired in the care you took of her and literally nobody else could have kept her going so long.' I reach the bottom, turn and find his hand held out and his face all puckered, just breaking into tears. I shake it hurriedly – make off and call back that I will wait to hear from him as to news. (I'll have to give medical evidence.) This is a poignant letter but I know you want the truth as it hits me.

March 29

Slept like a rock for the first time since I had 'flu, till 5.45. Am so thankful I took courage in both hands and went over to see Leonard yesterday. After a night of absorption of facts – the only way my slow brain works – I am now sure that, as long as war was on, I don't think it would have been possible to hold Virginia's mind. Without war I'm sure I could have helped and completely saved her. Tragic. Anyhow I'm also feeling today that I'm amazingly lucky to have had even that small amount of closeness to such a mind. But I do regret that I was not myself more warm and expressive, shall I say? But I never am – however I may feel, as you well know. Am afraid of it, I suppose? The last day we sat in that little room and I told her about my difficulties and about wanting to do Medicine, my moral cowardice and not daring to have it out with my family – about how I'd always lied to save my skin as a child, what it meant to meet you with your high standards, how you had made me feel so differently about Truth and so on. She sitting and interjecting helpful questions, sitting close to and hugging the fire – behind her that large window which overlooks the wide expanse of field and valley, flat and green, through which runs that evil river, which a week later was to clutch that free spirit (yes *indeed* free, if ever there was one, when the devil did not take possession) and which now is being dragged and won't give up its jealously held treasure.

To go back to my visit. I have a patient waiting this end at 6.15, the siren goes in the distance. It strikes me as remote and wholly of another world. Where that keen mind presided, Hitler, Luftwaffe and all the rest just did not exist. But my eye catches the clock. It's 6.10. 'Golly, I've a patient at 6.15.'

'Yes,' she looks up, her habit was to leave me her profile and only occasionally face me with a direct question; I'd taken this as her sensitiveness to my shyness in talking lamely about myself. 'Yes, but it's far more important for you to sit and talk to me,' and with a note of appeal, 'Don't go yet.' You will remember that when we went over together she always begged you not to go so soon. As I see it now, that contact with another and especially outside mind was a handrail that helped her. So I stay put, divided and tortured as usual between two loyalties – longing to stay and knowing the patient would be waiting. And in the interval (I don't recollect how it came out) but I say, looking out of the south window on my right, 'You have no idea how much I enjoy coming over, how it helps talking to an outsize mind.' And then, feeling desperate at my inability to find words, 'Oh, I can't say what I want,' and with my 'flu starting and a head of wool I subside sulkily into silence and wish for you as spokesman. She stirs and alters her position and says quietly: 'Oh, but do try – I want to know. You don't know how much I need it,' and eyes me gravely and steadily. I (again as usual) feel she is doing this to try to help my inadequacy with words. I had already told her that nothing [that] ever happened to me or was said to me sank in at the time and was only absorbed afterwards at its true value and she had been most understanding as to this. An easy person to talk with and a heavenly agility of mind which returned, as a first-class tennis player does, the most erratic or difficult ball. And now I realise I might have helped her – perhaps – quite considerably if I'd had the key to her need. As we went downstairs she says, 'Isn't there anything I can do for you? Can't I catalogue your books?' I say something grateful and in my own mind discard this idea as wholly improvident – would one employ a diamond cutter to hew coal? But if I'd known – it might have helped to give her such a manual job to keep the Beast at bay. Oh well, how I go on, to make you feel my every thought. Anyhow, apart from the personal sense of failure, did I tell you that in my reassurance to her on Thursday I'd said, 'There's nobody in England I want more to help than you.' And Leonard said that that evening, after her visit here, she was cheerful and quite different. Next day, alas! came the voices – the thing she had had before which always presaged disaster. Well, apart from my sense of being asked to get at it too late, I do feel now that short of end of war, I'd no hope of success.

N.B. Let us be realistic. If I'd had her here to do books and thought I was succeeding and then – this. Wouldn't it have been even worse?

On 19 April comes the following news which I quickly wrote to E.R.:

On Thursday night I dreamed so vividly that Virginia had turned up again, alive. So when I woke I was quite disappointed to know it was a dream. While I was out at Backset that evening Leonard rang and left me a message. Would I please ring him. This was to say they'd at last recovered the body and the inquest was yesterday. The Coroner apparently didn't need me. I'm glad it is now all over. One goes on regretting the waste. And quite plainly she was writing her very *best*. What tricks the mind was playing her. Also, how impossible it must be for a writer to judge his own work. Wasn't it odd that I'd dreamed of her like that? There's a lot we don't understand in this world.

At the beginning of August I drove over to see Leonard. Both E.R. and I were very anxious that he should publish Virginia's diaries which, at that time, he could not make up his mind to do. He was reluctant because there was too much about living people and because he felt it would give the wrong impression of her as a hypersensitive and moody person tormented by fears. He knew that for so much of the time she was an especially happy, gay, carefree person. I suggested that he should edit them where the 'moodiness' seemed to take charge, but this he said would not be honest. He felt they should be published fifty years hence and leave judgment to posterity. I pleaded the value of her methods to the new generation. He cited Katherine Mansfield, saying that no one had made the tears run down his cheeks with laughter as she had done in talk, and yet her Journals, edited by Murray, had given

an entirely different and false impression. We talked on about
Virginia and he told me how she would go to him with all her
difficulties, to 'have a thorn removed' as she always called it.
He said that for twenty-five years she had been struggling at
times with depressions and that he himself had had little idea
how continuous had been the battle. She wrote endlessly in her
diary and he had never known anyone so haunted and hurt
by criticism – not from knowledgeable critics only, but from
ignorant and inferior minds who knew nothing of writing. 'She
always wrote objectively,' he said, 'but she lived her life too
subjectively. She had, as I often told her, too ego-centric a
mind.' We talked a little more about the Diaries and then
Leonard said, 'We'd planned the next three books'; and he
spoke of the first two ideas and then added, 'We thought we'd
publish *Monday or Tuesday*, leaving out one story which she
thinks, and I agree, is bad.' His use of the present tense gave
me the feeling that he was conscious of Virginia's presence, as
if she'd just gone into a Room of her Own.

EPILOGUE

E.R. returned from America as early as possible after the Armistice in May 1945. She flew in a converted bomber which landed her in Ireland. She was then eighty-three years of age and her courage high as ever, but the journey was tiring and England not as she had expected. The domestic situation had changed, servants had almost vanished and food was still rationed. Her luggage, which she had sent by sea, took a long time to arrive, and she was anxious to continue the writing of her impressions of America under war conditions. When at last we heard that the steamer had arrived, we learned that practically everything she had brought back and valued most was rifled on the docks at Liverpool. We spent weeks over enquiries and advertisements but all to no avail. Her writings were lost. It was a time of short supply of paper. The railway paid up the value of other things, but nothing could recompense her for her work. It was a mortal blow. It broke her heart and made her feel that even England's high moral values had sunk. While she was in the United States she had been gravely shocked and discouraged by a fall when she broke her pelvis. She had suffered, out of all proportion, from the indignities and discomforts of hospital treatment in a country where she now felt herself an alien. Without the ceaseless care and devotion of the Henry Jameses she would, I felt from her letters, not have come through. She fretted to return to England, but this she was not allowed to do until the end of the war.

For the next few years she made my house in Montpelier Crescent her headquarters. She did a little writing and sorting of her belongings, and paid visits to some of the old friends who still remained. But she never really adapted herself to the combination of post-war conditions in England and her own increasing limitations. One of her favourite visitors was Leonard Woolf. She found his company very stimulating, he made her feel that she still had a part in literary life and she always looked forward to seeing him. Sybil Thorndike and Lewis Casson, too, used to visit her and through them she could keep abreast of the theatrical world.

My own work took up much time, and preparation for the National Health Service involved endless consideration. In 1948 it was introduced and I was put on to the Brighton and Lewes Hospital Management Committee. As the only representative of the New Sussex Hospital, it required both care and patience to see that the individuality and tradition of that institution was maintained.

In 1951 E.R. had a compelling urge to go back to her Eliot cousins in Pittsburgh for a short visit, in order to obtain a new brace for her back. She had a blind faith in a particular instrument-maker there. Dr Martindale was going over to a Medical Women's International Conference in Canada, and they valiantly flew off together in August to New York. On the way back they attended the United Nations at Lake Success and were greatly interested. Shortly after her return E.R. had another severe fall from which she never fully recovered, and six months later, on 8 May 1952, she died. After over forty years of close association, during which time I had referred all my happenings, whether good or ill, to her standard of what was right, the loss could have been unsupportable. Fortunately, my work at that time made exceptional claims.

By 1954 I was officially retired and could devote more time to Backsettown which became my headquarters. Backset had gone through a difficult time at the beginning of the war. We were in the invasion area in 1941 and had to get special police permits before our convalescents were allowed to come. We dispensed with the Matron, all nurses were desperately needed, and [instead we] found Mrs Vera Scott, who had run her own hotel at Whyteleaf until it was bombed. Backset has been endlessly grateful for her initiative, drive, gift for organisation and marvellous cooking. I still saw a few patients from time to time at Backset, and I could give a great deal more attention to my

Jersey herd. One day I was amazed when a farmer neighbour put my name forward, as a member of the Steyning National Farmers Union, to go on to the West Sussex County Council. At first I refused, but he urged me to think it over and, remembering how much my father enjoyed his work on the County Council, I finally agreed. Work on the County Council has been a most refreshing experience, and sometimes in sharp contrast to committees in the early days of the National Health Service, when there might be decidedly acrimonious discussions as to policy and the interpretation of the Act. Doctors have not always the most flexible minds, and we tend to be dogmatic. On the County Council Committees I was immediately struck by the courteous, good-tempered approach and the urgent desire of members to ensure that the right and sensible line of action should be taken for the welfare of West Sussex.

Much has been said and written about retirement. I have always remembered the words of an American physician dealing with the years from sixty to ninety. He points out the compensations that offset waning capacities of bone and muscle by enlarging powers of thought and opportunity for meditation. 'Creativeness in the realm of thought,' says Dr George Draper, 'has often reached its highest expression at this period, and wisdom, which is perhaps the greatest faculty of the human mind, finds here its fullest growth.' It is not so many years since women in the middle age group donned a lace cap and resigned themselves to a life of boredom when their children no longer needed their care. In these days, a woman can find her middle years the time of her greatest creative achievement. E.R. had felt this strongly and wrote in her diary on her fifty-sixth birthday: 'Anybody can be a successful young person. Youth is in itself accepted as success. To be a successful old woman – that's the great achievement.'

One day during August I was in London, the rain was pelting relentlessly down, and I sought refuge in Westminster Abbey. My feet carried me, almost automatically, to William Wilberforce's monument and I crouched to read, once again, the inscription on the base of the tomb. I sat for a while thinking about William. He had always had a respect and admiration for the abilities of women. He lived to see the realisation of his own dream of freedom for the enslaved peoples, as I have seen, in my lifetime, women's emancipation from most of their shackles. With the passing of the Married Women's Property Act they were allowed to own and control their own money; with the passing of the Women's Suffrage Bill, they were given a political vote. A hundred years ago women were not allowed to study for a medical degree. Thirteen years ago the elected candidate for the Presidency of the Royal College of Obstetrics and Gynaecology was a woman, Dame Hilda Lloyd. In my own practice I had always considered that T.B. meningitis was the most fell of all diseases, one which seemed to strike at the cleverest, most attractive child in a family and which was inexpressibly pitiable to watch in its tragically downward path. Now it is curable and I rejoice in the fact that a woman was responsible for the imagination and initiative which brought about its cure. These are but a few of countless examples of the work of women.

In my youth education for girls in England was not generally accepted as essential to their background. In the middle classes the main object was for parents to bring up their daughters to be sufficiently attractive to gain a suitable husband, to produce large families and be accomplished in the art of managing servants and the entertainment of guests. If they failed to marry they might become governesses or settle down to being 'old maids'. Equal opportunity in education, as in many other spheres of life, is now open to women, and the benefits of birth control and family planning, which ensure better health for both children and mothers, have proved infinite. In spite of acute domestic problems, the increase in the pace of life and of nuclear explosions, I have a profound belief in the contribution woman can make in the construction, as against destruction, of lives in the world. Indeed, my hope in the future lies in the exertions of women to bring a balance into world affairs, to conserve, construct, create, and this with no detriment to beauty, for 'a quickening of the motions of the mind will light a lamp behind the mask of beauty which makes it shine as it never shone before'.

Index

Index